"*The Queen of Distraction* strikes gold! It is the mother lode of wisdom, practical nuggets, humor, and insight. Terry Matlen is a true veteran of the ADHD saga. This book is authoritative, yet warm; up-to-date, yet timeless. Terry's masterful guide will help you feel less stressed, more successful, and happier in pursuit of your goals. I recommend it most highly."

—**Edward Hallowell, MD**, coauthor of *Driven to Distraction* and *Delivered from Distraction*

"*The Queen of Distraction* is an oasis of acceptance and practical ideas for women with ADHD—compassionate and approachable."

—**Melissa Orlov**, author of *The Couple's Guide to Thriving with ADHD*

"As a woman who suffers from ADHD herself, Matlen has personally walked the talk. Professionally, she's worked with countless others with adult ADHD through her coaching and consulting practice. Matlen's new book serves as an ADHD primer and introduction to all things ADHD. Keep it by your bedside, handy for when you feel low, confused, or alone. Terry's warm, knowledgeable voice will shine through like a beacon, guiding you with a voice that is supportive and accepting, knowledgeable and practical. Use it as a roadmap and companion as you navigate your journey with adult ADHD."

—**Zoë Kessler, BA, BEd**, author of *ADHD According to Zoë*

"Terry has done an exceptional job bringing together what is known about the science of attention deficit/hyperactivity disorder (ADHD) in adults as it applies specifically to women, making it live with numerous case examples of women with ADHD telling their own personal stories, and chock-full of sound advice for how to manage the symptoms, deficits, and impairments that are often associated with this disorder in adults. It is among the best and certainly the most current book on the topic of women with ADHD and will be exceptionally valuable to not only women with the disorder but those wishing to better understand it. It is certainly a must-read for therapists and coaches who assist such women through their practices."

—**Russell A. Barkley, PhD**, clinical professor of psychiatry
and pediatrics at Medical University of South Carolina,
RussellBarkley.org and ADHDLectures.com

"*The Queen of Distraction* is a must-read book for understanding how to deal with all the critical problems women with ADHD face daily. It is an appealing, practical, and easy-to read book written with insight, humor, and honesty. The real-life stories and examples provide the optimism and motivation to use the work/life tips to overcome ADHD-related challenges. Matlen provides a gift to women with ADHD. If the goal is managing difficulties such as transitions, clutter, time, emotions, relationships, or parenting, then Matlen provides a critical guide to greater productivity and life satisfaction."

—**Geraldine Markel, PhD**

"Terry Matlen has learned the hard way how to live a good life with ADHD. Fortunately for her readers, she is smart and funny enough that they can benefit from her experience and wisdom. She does an excellent job of explaining how ADHD impacts the specific demands women face today and offering solutions to make their lives better. This book will make your life easier—you need it!"

—**Ari Tuckman, PsyD, MBA**, author of *Understand Your Brain, Get More Done*; *More Attention, Less Deficit*; and *Integrative Treatment for Adult ADHD*

"Like most of my colleagues, I read each ADHD book that comes out, comparing the usefulness of one to the other. Terry Matlen has hit it out of the ballpark with this one. From the unique and relatable cover, which hints at humor, yet promises content, Ms. Matlen delivers to the reader a most thorough and *helpful* handbook for living inside a female, ADHD body (my personal favorite chapter: 'Clothing Loathing'). Not only does this book lighten the guilt of how we all feel in our clutter, chaos, and 'lack of measuring up' to Sally Struthers next door, it also takes each symptom and breaks it down into practical, easy steps to living a more productive and *comfortable* life! What a concept! Bravo to Matlen for this treasure, which will no doubt become the most worn-out book in any woman's ADHD library."

—**Wilma Fellman, MEd, LPC**, career counselor, ADHD coach and trainer, and author of *Finding a Career That Works for You* and *The Other Me: Poetic Thoughts on ADD for Adults, Kids and Parents*

"Terry Matlen gives the royal treatment to the topic of women with ADHD in her new book, *The Queen of Distraction*. Weaving together a combination of stories from her professional work and her own experience of living with ADHD, Matlen takes readers through all the struggles confronted by women with ADHD in today's world and provides useful coping tips for tackling them. Whether you are a woman with ADHD or you want to understand the impact of ADHD on the life of your mother, sister, daughter, partner, or any other woman in your life, this book is for you."

> **—J. Russell Ramsay, PhD**, associate professor of clinical psychology in psychiatry, codirector of the Adult ADHD Treatment and Research Program at the Perelman School of Medicine, University of Pennsylvania, and author of *The Adult ADHD Tool Kit*

"Many books offer advice to adults with ADHD about how they might cope more effectively with difficulties of daily life. This book is unique in its empathic understanding of emotional needs and stresses of women with ADHD who struggle to manage the complex demands of their daily life. It offers many very practical suggestions from an understanding friend who has been there and has learned from her experience."

> **—Thomas E. Brown, PhD**, associate director, Yale Clinic for Attention & Related Disorders, Yale University School of Medicine, and author of *Smart but Stuck: Emotions in Teens and Adults with ADHD*

"It's a fact! Women with ADHD are overwhelmed and hurting. Dial 911 and along comes Terry Matlen's *The Queen of Distraction* to the rescue, offering a prescription to help these women overcome chaos, clutter, and other everyday challenges. Like a skilled surgeon, Matlen cuts to the core of the problem and offers relief. I would recommend this book to every woman with ADHD. It doesn't matter whether she has an acute issue needing immediate attention or a chronic problem, is newly diagnosed or an 'old timer' looking for practical tips: help can be found within these pages."

—**Patricia O. Quinn, MD**, Center for Girls and Women
with ADHD, Washington, DC

"Every woman with ADHD should be issued a copy of *Queen of Distraction*. Written with compassion, wit, and brilliance and filled with practical ideas and encouragement—this is a must-have book for women with ADHD. However, as an ADHD coach, *The Queen of Distraction* is bad for business as she shares way too many strategies! There is probably well over two thousand dollars' worth of ideas, strategies and support for women with ADHD in these pages if you were to hire a coach. What a wonderful resource with women with ADHD.

"If you are a woman with ADHD, this book will soon become your new best friend. Anytime you are in need of understanding, support, encouragement, or help with practical strategies, this will become your go-to book over and over again."

—**Michele Novotni, PhD**, ADHD coach and author of
What Does Everybody Else Know that I Don't?

The

Queen

of

Distraction

How **Women**
with ADHD
Can Conquer Chaos,
Find Focus, *and*
Get More Done

TERRY MATLEN, MSW

New Harbinger Publications, Inc.

Distributed in Canada by Raincoast Books

Copyright © 2014 by Terry Matlen
        New Harbinger Publications, Inc.
        5674 Shattuck Avenue
        Oakland, CA 94609
        www.newharbinger.com

Cover design by Amy Shoup
Text design by Michele Waters-Kermes
Acquired by Melissa Valentine
Edited by Jean Blomquist

Library of Congress Cataloging-in-Publication Data

Matlen, Terry, 1953-
  The queen of distraction : how women with ADHD can conquer chaos, find focus, and get more done / Terry Matlen, MSW ; foreword by Sari Solden, MS LMFT.
    pages cm
  Includes bibliographical references.
  ISBN 978-1-62625-089-5 (paperback) -- ISBN 978-1-62625-090-1 (pdf e-book) -- ISBN 978-1-62625-091-8 (epub) 1. Attention-deficit disorder in adults--Popular works. 2. Women--Mental health--Popular works. 3. Attention-deficit disordered adults--Life skills guides. 4. Women--Life skills guides. 5. Mothers--Life skills guides. I. Title.
  RC394.A85M357 2014
  616.85'89--dc23
                      2014015747

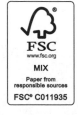
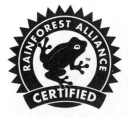

Printed in the United States of America

16   15   14

10 9 8 7 6 5 4 3 2 1   First printing

To the loves of my life:
Jerry, my husband
Kate and Mackenzie, my daughters
and Helen, my mother
…who make me laugh, cry, and everything in between.
How I cherish you!

Contents

Foreword

For the past twenty years I have had the great pleasure of knowing Terry Matlen professionally and personally, as her mentor and colleague. I have watched her become a respected and influential leader in the field of adults with ADHD and one of the handful of experts in the country who understands the special challenges and experiences of women with ADHD. Terry has accomplished this through her pioneering online work, writing, work with the media, memberships on boards of national ADHD organizations, and through her coaching and presentations.

On a personal level, Terry openly and generously shares her own experiences with ADHD with her audiences, readers, and clients. This personal wisdom and professional knowledge informs all of her work and allows her to convey the nuances and subtleties of the experience of women with ADHD. Far from giving formulaic advice, Terry's new book combines her thirst for research with her understanding of the inner, felt experience of this group of women.

I met Terry when I was writing my book, *Women with Attention Deficit Disorder*, which was originally published in 1995 (new edition, 2005). Women with this unique brain chemistry and life experience reported that, in reading the book, they were able to see their most secret experiences described in detail for the first time. It unleashed a wave of excitement in these readers as well as professional interest about this group of typically undiagnosed women who didn't fit the stereotype of hyperactive boys that prevailed at the time. As a psychotherapist, I focused on what happens to women who aren't able to meet gender role expectations due to their challenges. I explored the resulting shame and guilt that keeps them from moving toward their strengths, their dreams, and a fulfilling life.

This is the experience, perspective, and lens through which I read what is written for and about women with ADHD. Often books, articles, or presentations for these women focus only on the symptoms that can be observed from the outside or on strategies that aren't connected to or don't take into account the internal experiences that are so intimately intertwined with their challenges. As a result, women seeking help are often set up for frustration and failure. Terry's new book, *The Queen of Distraction*, adds the missing pieces by connecting her excellent strategies to the inner experience of the reader while recognizing that employing these strategies is much more complex than simply buying a fancy new planner or taking medication.

Terry provides detailed descriptions of and solutions for areas of high impact for women with ADHD, such as shopping, dressing, and managing clutter. Despite a clear recognition of these issues, her writing has no hint of subtle blaming, shaming, or stereotyping but is instead infused with respect for the struggle. She is able to communicate the important truth that women with ADHD must not define themselves by their challenges.

Terry brings all this to life through her humor, memorable stories of real women with ADHD, and a warm, inviting tone that helps women feel understood and accepted. Her personal honesty is extremely therapeutic. Her openness gives women who have long lived with ADHD in secret permission to accept themselves in the same way Terry has learned to do. The reader comes to feel the sense of belonging and understanding that is often missing from her life.

The Queen of Distraction is comprehensive but extremely well organized in a format that is easy for women with ADHD to read, absorb, and identify with. It goes beyond simple solutions, definitions, diagnoses, and stereotypes to present an authentic, accurate view with a fresh, original approach. Terry's metaphor of triage in various areas of challenge, such as dealing with clutter, is especially compelling and intriguing and a useful way to prioritize and take needed action.

Whether you are newly diagnosed or a woman who has been diagnosed for years, I highly recommend you read this book all the way through. After that, keep it close by to refer to when you need a great personal coach like Terry right there beside you. Equally important, though, open it whenever you feel overwhelmed or vulnerable—when you need a reminder, as we all do from time to time, that your struggles are real, that they originate in your brain, that they are not reflections of your character or your personal failings, and that there are countless other women who share this journey with you.

—Sari Solden, MS, LMFT

Acknowledgments

This book would not have seen the light of day had it not been for Melissa Valentine and the team at New Harbinger Publications. Thank you for finding me and putting your faith in me. Many thanks go to my writing coach and editor, Jeannie Ballew of Edit Prose, who stuck with me through thick and thin and helped make my words shine brightly. I couldn't have done this without your expert help and gentle, kind support.

I'd also like to thank Sari Solden, whose groundbreaking work in the field of women with ADIID inspired me to choose this path of helping others with ADHD. I will always be grateful for your generous support and encouragement.

I'd also like to thank all of you who have reached out to me over the years, sharing your stories, your heartbreaks, and your successes. I've learned so much from you. You are such an inspiration—do not ever lose hope!

To my dear mother, Helen Wachler, who told me on a daily basis while writing this book how proud she was of me—even at my age! I was lucky to have been raised by a mother who embraced creative thinking and expression and who told me I could succeed in whatever path I chose, regardless of the grades on my report cards. And to my stepfather, Norman Wachler, for the stability he gave our family and the wisdom that he shared throughout the years.

To my unique and wonderful daughters, Kate and Mackenzie, thank you for being my shining stars. There are no words to express my love for you. You make my life a complete joy!

And to my dearest husband, Jerry—my rock, best friend, and fishing buddy—thank you for your patience, support, and belief in me, and for keeping me afloat this past year while my head was in this book. Thank you for your unwavering love, your ability to make me laugh hysterically even after all these years…and the hundreds of carryout dinners that thankfully found their way to the table.

Introduction

I have been in your shoes. I lived with undiagnosed ADHD for over forty years.

When my kids were little, figuring out what to make for dinner each night—and pulling it off—felt like an Olympian challenge. I faced piles of laundry because I struggled to decipher the seemingly simple steps of sorting, washing, drying, and putting it away. It was typical to wake up to a wet heap of smelly clothes in the washer because I had forgotten to load the dryer the night before. I avoided talking on the phone because, if I couldn't see the speaker's mouth, I couldn't focus on the words, and my mind would drift a hundred miles away. My house was cluttered, bills were paid late, and, over and over, I asked myself, *How can I earn two academic degrees but not be able to file ten papers? What is wrong with me?*

Discovering that I had ADHD and getting help for it changed my life in ways I never dreamed possible. As I gained confidence in myself through learning more about ADHD and how it affected me, I began to baby-step my way into a new, exciting life that included this thing called ADHD. I learned that my ADHD didn't define me but explained many of my quirks and difficulties. Once I saw how vastly different—and better—my life became, I wanted to offer hope to other women with ADHD, women like you who might be living in shame, self-loathing, or pure frustration.

Since the mid-1990s, I have been working with adults with ADHD in a variety of capacities. I volunteered for many years at CHADD (Children and Adults with Attention-Deficit/Hyperactivity Disorder) and ADDA (Attention Deficit Disorder Association). I led support groups online and launched http://ADDconsults.com, where I've been able to meet and help thousands of men and women online. My journey led me to writing my first book, *Survival Tips for Women with ADHD*. Who would have thought that the quiet, sensitive soul who was happiest locked up in a cozy room reading a book would end up presenting talks to hundreds of people around the country on the topic of women with ADHD?

My hope is that this book will continue my voyage toward helping other women with ADHD who, like me, got so very stuck with the symptoms of ADHD: drowning in clutter, being late, burning dinner, feeling constantly overwhelmed. I'm living proof that you can move on despite your ADHD and find happiness and success. No, it's not a walk in the park. It takes lots of hard work and perseverance. But it *can* be done.

I hope this book will help you start your own journey and that you will find that your ADHD is only a small part of who you are. The information and tips that follow will help you get started on your way to becoming the person you were meant to be. After all, she's been there all along.

A Note to Readers: Throughout the book, I will be using masculine pronouns for partners. This is for convenience only; I do not intend to exclude readers with same-sex partners.   —TM

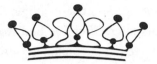

CHAPTER 1

What the Heck Is ADHD, Anyway?

Best friends since nursery school, Liz and Alex liked to refer to themselves as sisters, though they couldn't have been more different. Liz was tall, dark, thin, and brooding, whereas Alex was short, athletic, cheerful, and constantly in motion. They are now in their early thirties. Over the years, Alex juggled multiple low-paying jobs while performing at local theater and musical festivals on the weekends. She got fired from job after job due to poor performance, not getting projects done on time, being late almost daily, or not getting along with coworkers. Liz, on the other hand, felt constantly overwhelmed by teaching and her two highly active children.

One fall weekend, Liz and Alex drove to a cottage in Canada, deliriously happy to escape their troubles even if just for a few days. Upon arrival, Liz parked herself in a hammock near the beach with a novel and promptly fell asleep. When she awoke, Alex was nowhere to be found. Liz's head filled with worst-case scenarios: *Maybe she got swept up in the waves. Could there be bears? Maybe she got lost!* She tried calling Alex's cell, but Alex didn't answer. Hours later, after Liz had worked herself into a tizzy, Alex came barreling through the screen door, grinning from ear to ear, and launched into how she'd seen a fox, snapping turtles, lizards, and more on her nature adventure. When Liz glared at her and told her how sick with fear she'd been, Alex stopped dead in her tracks. Once again, she'd failed a friend with her impulsive ways. They sat down, had a heart-to-heart, and put it behind them. Well, Alex did. But Liz spent the next hour ruminating over her friend's apparent lack of courtesy and worried how their weekend together was going to pan out.

Do either of these women's behaviors sound familiar? Alex is full of fun and adventure, constantly on the move, slamming through life like a hurricane, leaving crumpled papers and relationships in her path. Liz feels everything with intensity and worries over details; she is often lost in her rich, dreamy internal world, escaping to it frequently while life goes whizzing by her. She is easily distracted, leaving a trail of unfinished projects behind her that give clues as to her latest interests and activities. Maybe you, like both Alex and Liz, have adult ADHD (attention deficit/hyperactivity disorder). In this chapter, we will review our current understanding of ADHD, the different subtypes, and the various terms that have been used for it in the past.

The Nuts and Bolts of ADHD

Attention deficit/hyperactivity disorder (ADHD) is a *neurobiological disorder*—in other words, a disorder in the biology of the nervous system—characterized by impairment of executive functions and self-regulation. This results in inattention, hyperactivity/impulsivity, or a combination of the two. In order for a diagnosis of ADHD to be made, the disorder has to have started in childhood and cause impairment for the individual in one or more environments (work, home, and so on). Let's look more closely at the results of impairments in executive functioning.

Who among us hasn't had trouble composing that first sentence for a paper or an important letter? It's not easy, but many of us do eventually get past the mental impasse and summon the complex planning and organizational skill necessary to write term papers, run work projects, plan a kitchen renovation, or separate dark-colored laundry from light. *Executive function* (EF) is an imposing name for a group of essential mental tasks that help us achieve those goals:

- planning

- strategizing

- organizing

- goal setting

- paying attention to important details

Executive functioning, the control panel of your brain, basically involves figuring out how to get from step A to step B to step C. It is like the track that keeps the train on course as it stops, starts, and turns, getting you to your destination.

In addition to poor executive functioning, ADHD involves poor self-regulation. According to internationally recognized ADHD expert Dr. Russell Barkley (2013), adults with ADHD typically:

- become easily distracted by stimuli

- find it hard to stop behaviors and activities that are engaging and of interest to them

- impulsively make decisions

- don't follow directions carefully when starting a project

- often don't follow through on promises or commitments

- have trouble doing things in proper sequence

- speed while driving

- find it hard to enjoy quiet leisure activities

These symptoms exemplify how impairing ADHD can be to a woman because they encompass just about all the facets of her life. Though "executive functioning" and "self-regulation" sound like terminology straight out of a college textbook, suffice it to say that these seemingly "absentminded" behaviors are, in fact, *brain* based, and there is a perfectly rational explanation for why you "do the things you do."

Introducing the ADHD Subtype Trio

ADHD (commonly called ADD, or attention deficit disorder) is an umbrella term that encompasses the three subtypes of ADHD. Though the vast majority of cases of ADHD are genetic, in some cases, one can *acquire* ADHD through brain injury, illness, or prenatal exposure to toxic substances. It is important to note that ADHD is *not* caused by poor parenting, excessive TV, or one's diet.

Though neither Alex nor Liz has officially been diagnosed with ADHD, they exhibit classic symptoms. We'll explore their symptoms a bit more below after a discussion of the three subtypes of ADHD:

- hyperactive/impulsive

- inattentive

- combined

The most common is the combined subtype, which, as the name suggests, combines both hyperactive/impulsive and inattentive symptoms. Let's go through each subtype and look at some of the common symptoms seen in each.

Hyperactive/Impulsive Subtype

Hyperactive/impulsive subtype behavior is characterized by incessant mental, verbal, or physical activity that is often carried out without consideration of consequences. Typically, these behaviors are less overt in adults than they are during childhood. Answer these questions, and see if you exhibit any of the behaviors or tendencies they describe:

- Do you have a hard time finishing a book?

- Do you fidget during meetings, tapping your fingers or swinging your feet?

- Do you blurt out things and interrupt others, or have you been told that you simply talk too much?

- Do you find it hard to relax?

- Do you enjoy high-stimulation activities even if they might be dangerous?

- Do you overeat, overspend, over-everything?

- Do you leave a trail of "stuff" everywhere?

- Do you sometimes feel out of step socially?

Though all adults have some of these problems, an adult with ADHD will have them more frequently and find them to be troublesome in life. If you have many of these problems and they interfere with your life, it may be time to get an evaluation for ADHD.

Inattentive Subtype

The woman with the inattentive subtype of ADHD often lives a quieter, more internal life than her hyperactive/impulsive countertype. She is prone to daydreaming, feels a chronic sense of being overwhelmed, and worries and ruminates. Inattentive women may be physically sluggish or prefer quiet activities, but many have hyperactive brains that crave stimulation as well. It's important to understand that both subtypes have symptoms in common. See if you answer yes to a majority of the questions below that describe common symptoms seen in adults with the inattentive subtype of ADHD:

- Do you have trouble paying attention to detail?

- Do you make careless mistakes?

- Do you tend to be shy?

- Do you feel sluggish much of the time?

- Do you struggle with hypersensitivities?

- Do you have trouble staying on task (unless it's an activity in which you have keen interest)?

- Do you have a poor memory?

- Do you see people's lips moving but don't pay attention to what they are saying?

- Do you often have difficulties following or understanding instructions?

- Do you avoid tasks that involve a lot of effort?

- Are you easily distracted?

- Do you forget where you've put things?

We all misplace our keys or fade out of a boring conversation at times. If, however, you have many of the symptoms above and they impair your life to some degree, it's time to be evaluated for possible inattentive ADHD.

Combined Subtype

A woman with the combined subtype of ADHD has symptoms of both inattention *and* hyperactivity/impulsivity, but not enough inattentive or hyperactivity/impulsivity symptoms to warrant a diagnosis of either of those subtypes. She may be constantly on the run but also have a dreamy quality to her personality, getting lost in her thoughts and missing the finer details in her work and life in general.

It's important to note that there is a paucity of studies attempting to describe the subtypes of ADHD in adults, and symptoms of all three subtypes may overlap. But knowing what subtype you might have can help you and your therapeutic team. For example, women with inattentive ADHD might be more prone to depression than their hyperactive/impulsive counterparts, so practitioners might be extra careful in looking for symptoms of depression that also need to be addressed.

Looking back at the Liz and Alex vignette, we can see that Liz has inattentive ADHD—she's dreamy, in her own world at times, distractible, and introverted—whereas Alex exemplifies the combined subtype, as she has symptoms of hyperactivity/impulsivity (dashing out into the lake) yet also has inattentive traits (not paying attention to Liz's feelings and needs). If you're a bit confused by this terminology soup, take heart—you're not alone. Even the experts can't agree on everything!

Is ADHD a Disease, a Condition, or a New Cable Channel?

ADHD has gone through so many different definitions that, after you've heard them all, you may ask, "Will the real definition please stand up?" These definitions have ranged from "minimal brain damage" to "hyperkinetic reaction of childhood or adolescence." At the turn of the twentieth century, doctors such as British pediatrician Sir George Frederick Still (1902) described children with ADHD-like symptoms as having a "moral defect." Later these children were thought to have suffered brain damage. In the 1960s, there began a shift toward thinking of this disorder as a behavioral syndrome with a biological basis. In the late 1970s, clinicians began to focus on the possibility that not just children but also adults could have ADHD, and in the 1980s, that focus shifted from just hyperactivity to deficits in attention (Lange et al. 2010). It is often now referred to as attention deficit/hyperactivity disorder (ADHD), though many simplify the terminology by calling it attention deficit disorder (ADD). Either is acceptable.

Just as experts have grappled with the terminology, so have they also tried to discern if ADHD is a neurobiological brain-based disorder, a disease, or a condition. A study published in the *Journal of Neuropsychiatry and Clinical Neurosciences* (Courvoisie et al. 2004) states that there are .

actual chemical differences between the ADHD brain and the non-ADHD brain. So whether it's a disorder, disease, or condition is a matter of semantics, but it's important to know that every person with ADHD is an individual with strengths and challenges. No two people with ADHD share the same exact symptoms.

In an effort to "make friends" with ADHD, some describe it as a "gift," but there haven't been any solid studies to prove that, and professional opinions are mixed. Dr. Russell Barkley (2010) rejects the notion that ADHD is a gift "or that it predisposes to anything positive in human life." ADHD expert Dr. Edward (Ned) Hallowell suggests in the biography page on his website that, rather than a disorder, ADHD is "a gift that is hard to unwrap," and he leans toward seeing ADHD as a condition that can be tamed so that one's true abilities, creativity, and gifts can shine through.

One ability or gift that often shines through is thinking outside the box. Many of us who work in the ADHD field notice that a good number of our clients do that naturally. That's not to say, however, that your ability to think outside the box or your ADHD is always an advantage. Often, it gets in the way of expressing your creativity. In the case of Alex, her ADHD got in the way of finding success in her music career. Her dream of forming her own band and writing original songs vanished. She just couldn't get along with others, nor could she finish what she started whenever she attempted to pen a new melody.

As researchers try to figure out what exactly ADHD is, it's clear that "attention deficit/hyperactivity disorder" is actually a misnomer because there isn't a *deficit* of attention but rather an inability to *control* it. You may not have the patience to file paperwork for more than ten minutes, but you can browse—read *hyperfocus*—on the Internet for two hours because it holds your interest. Some people even humorously call it attention *surplus* disorder because of how quickly you can change your attention from one thing to another, depending on what interests or distracts you. Attention can be scattered, diffuse, or laser-like, but rarely anything in between.

My own personal and professional leanings on what ADHD is tend to lie somewhere between Dr. Barkley's and Dr. Hallowell's definitions.

ADHD can be a disabling disorder, but with the proper treatment, many people can uncover their strengths and soar. The key is getting the appropriate help.

If you have not already been diagnosed, perhaps you're curious enough now to pursue an evaluation. If that's the case, you might wonder what to do first. My advice is to start by seeing your primary care physician or other health care provider and get a complete physical workup. You want to make sure that your symptoms can't be attributed to a physical cause, such as an under- or overactive thyroid, allergies, or a sleep disorder. If you've been medically cleared, then it's time to pursue an ADHD evaluation. Since adult ADHD, unfortunately, is still not well understood by many clinicians, it's to your advantage to find someone (psychiatrist, psychologist, neurologist, or other mental health professional) with expertise in adult ADHD. Too many adults, especially women, are misdiagnosed as having depression because many of those symptoms overlap with ADHD—or you might have depression in addition to your ADHD because your life has been filled with chaos, underperformance, and low self-esteem from repeated failures in certain areas of your life. Since ADHD rarely travels alone, there is a good chance you may have a coexisting condition, such as depression, anxiety, or addictive behaviors, that also needs to be addressed. That's why you want to find a professional who can sort these things out.

Treatment for adult ADHD typically includes medication (when recommended), counseling, education, support (for example, support groups), and ADHD coaching. ADHD coaching involves working on pragmatic life skills that are impaired by your ADHD. An ADHD coach works with you on such areas as time management, organizing, and procrastination, and helps you break old habits and learn new, healthier, and more effective strategies in these areas. You should get information and resources for all of these options from your clinician. If you're not sure you have ADHD and would like to learn more about getting a qualified diagnosis or exploring typical treatment options, you can find in-depth information about both diagnosis and treatment on my website at http://ADDconsults.com.

By getting diagnosed, being treated, and reading books like this one, you will begin to understand why you've struggled with many areas of your life. For example, one of the most frequent complaints I hear from women with ADHD is their struggle with clutter. But this isn't a character flaw, personality disorder, or weakness. It's simply a result of how your brain is wired. So let's jump right in and find out how to tame the "clutter beast."

CHAPTER 2

My Life Is Buried Under One of These Piles

Alex is cussing. Loudly. Annoyance escalates into rage as she stomps around her house searching for the letter to appear in court for a speeding ticket. Teeth clenched, she admonishes herself for not having put it in her new "to-do" folder. She calls the court and finds out that she missed her appointment and is now in danger of losing her license. Clutter: 1/Alex: 0. Again.

What exactly is clutter? For some, it's three pieces of mail sitting on the kitchen counter. For those of us with ADHD, it's three *feet* of paper someplace where it does not belong. Sadly, as a woman with ADHD, you might be defining your self-worth by how much clutter you have lying about your home or workspace or even in your car. It becomes your obsession, your nemesis; your daily reminder that your life is out of control, that you haven't mastered the art of maintaining your living area and workspace like everyone else has by the time they are sixteen. You've probably heard comments such as these your entire life: "Why can't she put her stuff away?" "Doesn't she care how it affects the rest of us?" "Why is she so lazy?" "What a pig!" And you have most likely internalized these painful, derogatory, negative remarks over the years until they have slaughtered your self-esteem, making you wonder *What is wrong with me?*

Clutter and chronic disorganization combine to create a virtual hellhole for women with ADHD, a seemingly endless abyss that threatens to suck them down on a daily basis. The compromised executive functioning of the ADHD brain makes all things weigh in as equally important, thereby making sorting, selecting, and tossing a real challenge. Though seemingly mundane tasks are extremely challenging for the woman with ADHD, if she is partnered or married with children, she is quite often expected, as the home manager, to manage not only her own mass of papers and personal belongings but also those of her children and spouse. This chapter offers insights into the underlying brain-based issues that contribute to clutter and disorganization, the resulting emotional issues that often go hand in hand with that clutter, and pragmatic, get-it-done solutions to help you manage the clutter beast and keep it in its cage.

What Does My Brain Have to Do with My Messy House?

Messiness. Clutter. Disorganization. These are not character flaws. They are symptoms of how your ADHD brain functions. The lack of executive functioning directly contributes to why it is so hard for you to stop the overflow of papers, toys, kitchen utensils, and clothing as they cascade from your kitchen table, desk, and closet onto the floor. Executive function impairment is universally seen in adults with ADHD. It's no mystery that your space is taken over by stuff because your brain has a hard time prioritizing *what* to do first, *how* to do it best, and *when* to do it. Your brain's circuitry finds it difficult to prioritize (*Do I pay the bill first or send in the wedding RSVP?*), stick with "boring" tasks (*Paperwork is so boring. I think I'll play a video game instead*), or sort (*Do I file it under "Car" or stick it in "Bills Paid"?*). Do you also have trouble starting or stopping a task? If so, you are not alone. Starting requires prioritizing and decision making.

Stopping is hard because once you get into a task, you may tend to hyper-focus and have time distortion—what seems like five minutes is actually thirty or vice versa—as well as difficulty transitioning from one activity to another. And on and on it goes. Think about the symptoms typically seen in ADHD that we talked about in chapter 1—impulsivity, inattention, procrastination, difficulty transitioning, and forgetfulness. Let's take a closer look at each of these now.

Impulsivity

You see something in the store and purchase it, not realizing at the time that you don't need it, don't have the space for it, or, worse, already have two of them. The outcome? The new item lands on a table and stays there for weeks, months, or longer, until you find the time to make a decision as to what to do with it. By then, you probably decide that you'd like to return it, but find that either you've lost the receipt or it's too late to take it back.

Inattention

As with impulsivity, you see something you like—shoes, for example—and purchase them, not realizing they don't remotely match anything in your closet. Or, at a garage sale, you snag a great bargain—the perfect dresser for storing all the things you seem to collect but have no room for—but you've forgotten that there is zero space in your house to put the dresser. Or you're so wrapped up in watching the *Morning Show* every Wednesday that you don't think to take out the garbage, and you now have three weeks' worth of trash stinking up your garage.

Procrastination

Clutter can also be a result of procrastination. It's right there, facing you eyeball to eyeball, reminding you of just how difficult it is to take care of your stuff. If you can't figure out where to put your things or find it too difficult or too boring to set up a system for your stuff and simply put off doing anything about it, there it lies, underfoot, sometimes forever.

Years ago, when I needed to set up my home office, I hired a professional organizer who taught me something so fundamental that I was shocked that I had never understood the concept before: *everything you own needs a home*. Once there's a home for everything, clutter becomes less of a problem. Clutter happens when you don't know what to do with things, or when you have duplicates of something you've forgotten you already own. By creating a home for each of your things, when you have an item in your hand that needs to be put away, you now have a place where it belongs.

Difficulty Transitioning

But here is another ADHD dilemma: being unable to transition from a pleasurable activity to an unpleasant task, like putting items away. For most women with ADHD, this is simply too boring to deal with, period. It's much more interesting to work on scrapbooking, play a computer game, or watch a movie than to declutter the house. And if your house is filled with distractions, it's a double whammy. Add a partner and/or kids, and the clutter builds up to tsunami proportions because your attention is pulled in so many directions.

Where Did I Put My Meds?
I Can't Remember!

As a woman with ADHD, you likely have a difficult time remembering where you've put something; or if you did put it away, you've forgotten where you stored it, since you no longer can see it. This brings us to what I call Clutter "Junky" Maxim #1: *Gotta see it to remember I have it!* Related to problems with working memory, if an item is out of sight, it's out of mind. But you were probably taught as a child that your belongings needed to be put away so that they would not be an eyesore. So you stuff things in boxes, closets, and drawers. Or you dump them on a flat surface using what I call a "horizontal filing system": piling things up until they spill east, west, north, and south. Welcome to the ADHD landslide!

Even if you have good intentions of managing your stuff, it may take a catastrophe, like not being able to find your passport for an upcoming trip, for you to decide that you *must* declutter your room. But then, how do you start? Do you just aimlessly begin filing papers, throwing stuff in boxes, or tossing things in the garbage? The whole mess becomes overwhelming to the point where you give up and hang your head in shame.

What Emotional Buttons Does Clutter Push?

If you have ADHD and especially if you haven't yet been adequately treated for it, then more than likely you have clutter. You probably grew up with clutter. Perhaps your bedroom always had a mass of clothes lying on the floor. Your toys were strewn throughout the house. Schoolwork was in piles on your desk. And chances are, your parents, siblings, and teachers criticized you for not being able to keep your stuff together in an organized fashion. Having heard negative comments about this for years, you probably associate your clutter with the words you heard growing up—words such as "lazy," "unmotivated," or "selfish." And worse.

Perhaps you grew up worried about what people thought of you. Perhaps your self-esteem took a hit, eventually leading to anxiety and depression. Did you wonder how you could, say, earn a college degree yet not be able to figure out how to organize your kitchen or closet? Your inner world reflects your external world: a life of chaos in which you experience anxiety every day because you can't find what you need. Or perhaps you overcompensated for your lack of innate tidiness by turning into a perfectionist. If so, what kind of emotional and physical toll has that taken on you?

911 for Mess Distress!

Dr. Martin Luther King Jr. said, "Take the first step in faith. You don't have to see the whole staircase—just take the first step." So let's break organizing clutter down into smaller steps. The next time you pick up a piece of paper, a kitchen tool, or any household object and find yourself struggling with where it belongs, ask yourself, *Where is the most logical place for this?* Its home should be where it is typically used. Oven mitts near the oven. Magazine clippings in a folder in your home office. Take the item and move it to that area and make a new home for it. Taking small steps like this will mitigate the agony of having to make a lot of decisions all at once about where to put things.

Clutter Triage

One of the most difficult things to do when faced with items that need to be put away and organized is determining where to start and how to prioritize. To simplify this common problem, let's refer to the medical triage concept of prioritizing actions based on the severity of the problem—for example:

A. Are you bleeding to death and need immediate assistance in order to survive as you're being rushed to the ER?

B. Do you have a serious health problem—like needing a liver transplant—that must be treated with either surgery or medication but can wait a few months?

C. Do you have a crooked nose, which is not life threatening, that can wait for reconstructive surgery?

Now let's look at your clutter from a triage point of view:

A. What papers or things do you need to organize immediately that will be a serious threat to your comfort or survival if you don't take care of them now or in the near future?

B. What things do you need to keep track of that are not urgent but important?

C. What clutter can keep for a while until you have more time or energy to deal with it?

So when you're wondering where to start, think in terms of finding and organizing the most important, "need to take care of now" items first—like the electric bill, rent/mortgage, or insurance documents, or materials needed for that presentation you're giving in a few days. Then once all of those items are in their proper "homes," you can move on to the pile of library books that needs to be returned so you don't incur a late fee. And last but not least, you can go through your canned goods and toss out items that have expired.

Most of the books and websites that promise to solve your clutter problem have dozens and dozens of solutions. In my experience as an ADHD expert, consultant, and writer, the word "clutter" or "organize" in a book title is guaranteed to make most women with ADHD reach for their checkbook, since they're always searching for the magic solution to their chronic problems in this area. Despite these good intentions, most of us miss the boat. The books give us great tips, but we still lack a deeper understanding of how to manage this problem at the emotional and physical level. A journey inward will give you insights, tools, and tips for managing your outward journey and keeping your clutter under control. Let us also remember that finding the right medication in the right dosage can help our brains work better to manage the clutter and be more organized.

Use the Wisdom of the Body to Help You Prioritize

In addition to using the clutter triage approach, you can also make prioritizing easier by simply learning to *listen* to your body. Ask yourself,

What aspect of my clutter is making me feel so awful? Is it the suitcase I've yet to unpack from my vacation three months ago? Is it the trail of paper that greets me as I enter my kitchen every day? Is it the rotting vegetables in the fridge?

You will find your way better if you listen to *yourself*, not the outside influences that you've internalized from your spouse, parents, sibs, teachers, friends, or bosses. Start with these questions: *Where does it hurt? What are my physical survival needs, and what are my emotional survival needs? What is more important? Having milk in the fridge so I and/or the kids can have breakfast tomorrow, or calling Aunt Renee and wishing her a belated happy birthday?* Stress finds its way into your body in physical ways via migraines, muscle tension, insomnia, upset stomachs, and more. So, if the sight of an unpacked suitcase makes you feel physically ill, that's your cue to address that chore sooner rather than later.

Now that the priorities have been considered, let's get down to the nitty-gritty of tips for dealing with clutter and disorganization. The idea is to avoid feeling anxious, stressed, sick, and depressed over your chaos. In order to do that, let's pinpoint areas of potential daily stress.

The Launching Pad and Survival Kit

Using the clutter triage concept, the topics and tips in the rest of this chapter are organized from most-stress-inducing to least-stress-inducing. For many, the most stressful time of day is getting out the door in the morning to go to work and/or, if you have kids, getting them off to school. To help keep order during the morning rush, develop a launching pad—a designated space—for each family member (including you) near the door where that person exits. Place each person's survival kit on the launching pad. A survival kit includes all the basics needed for the day. Your survival kit, for example, might include these items:

- cell phone

- keys

- purse

- glasses

- briefcase

- accessories such as scarves, umbrella, gloves

The children's survival kits might include these items:

- backpack

- books

- lunch

- snack

- accessories such as hats, scarves, boots, or mittens

Children with ADHD find using a launching pad to be extremely helpful. It's novel and fun, and it engages them visually and tactilely. Not only do they see the items, they have to pick them up, so it engages the senses of both sight and touch. When it comes to learning and remembering things, the more senses that are involved, the better. To manage potential school-related clutter, go through the backpack every day with your child to throw out old food, trash, or unnecessary items.

Coats 'n' Cubbies

I've found that a great way to make a launching pad for the entire family is to purchase an inexpensive coat rack along with a set of cubbies. Insert a basket within each cubby to help manage belongings; the basket holds each person's survival kit. As family members leave in the morning, they check their baskets for the items they need to take with them. When they return in the afternoon or evening, have them (and you!) get into a routine of putting everything back in their cubby basket and hanging their jackets and backpacks on the coat rack. School- or work-related objects go into the cubby. There may not be enough room for shoes and boots; if not, add a rubber runner on the floor beneath the coat rack or add a shoe rack nearby.

Charging Stations

A great addition to your launching pad area is a charging station. It stores your electronics neatly while charging them up. (And if you leave them there, you won't have to deal with kids—or parents!—texting, checking e-mail, and surfing the Internet at the dinner table.) There are a number of attractive charging stations to choose from. Some even have small drawers for extra keys and such, so the station could also hold your survival kit. Label drawers as needed, or consider using an attractive cup, bowl, or small platter to hold your survival kit items.

Plan to Succeed

Having a launching pad and survival kits for all is a great first step, but even better is planning your launch—that is, having the survival kits ready to go—the night before (if you're a night owl) or early in the morning (if you're a morning person). Make a checklist for you and any family member who might benefit from a reminder system. This will ensure that everyone has everything in their survival kits before walking out the door. Making lists on scraps of paper, however, creates more clutter, so it may be necessary to come up with different strategies. One of my clients, for example, swears by the Boogie Board, a small LCD slate with stylus that you can purchase online. (Google "Boogie Board" or find it at http://ADDconsults.com.) You can jot down reminders, lists, and messages, then simply push a button to erase. This is a great product for helping you (and family members) remember to put items in the survival kit each day. Since they come in a variety of colors, each person could select a different color. As kids get older, you can encourage them to write down their survival kit list themselves. To keep their interest, add small check boxes before each item on your children's Boogie Boards. Then, when they place each listed item in their survival kit, they can check off the box, showing it has been done. (Another option is to use a paper list.) Here are some other possible items to list on their Boogie Boards:

- lunch money

- books (list each one)

- papers to be signed

- notes, such as "Remember to ask your teacher about the field trip permission slip"

These reminder tools aren't just for helping you keep your launching pad loaded and survival kits ready for the day. They also help with just about anything, such as shopping lists, notes to family members, or phone messages.

Your Phone as a Mobile Office

Today's smartphones are also chock-full of organizing tools. The simple memo application can be used for tons of things, like keeping track of gifts that need to be purchased, clothes sizes, shopping lists, birthdays, or when to get the oil changed.

Take a Picture: Make It Stick

We know that visual cues are extremely helpful for those with ADHD. Since most smartphones have camera capabilities, you can use yours (or a camera) to take a photo of your launching pad—and of individual survival kits—as a visual reminder. The photos would include the typical items in your or your child's survival kit—for example, cell phone, car keys, and glasses for you; and homework, house key, and snack for your child. You can even print out the pictures and tape them up above the launching pad to help you remember what items need to be in which survival kit. Laminating the photos will, of course, offer longevity, which is especially helpful if there are young children involved. One elderly woman I know has a photograph of the medications she takes each morning and night. It's laminated and sitting next to her pill bottles. This helps her to stay organized and keep track of her meds. Such a strategy would work wonderfully for your family members who are taking medications. The visuals could help them remember what to take and when. Speaking of using visuals to stay organized, phone photos are also a great way to remember where you parked your car. Simply take a snapshot of the lot number or aisle and/or nearby landmarks, like signs or structures. You can use any of the visual strategies listed above to help keep you and your stuff organized.

There's a Reason It's Called Paper*work*

If there's one plea I hear the most from women with ADHD, it's "Please help me with the paperwork!" They need help with managing paper: bills, magazines, receipts, children's artwork, school papers, taxes, and the like. Doing paperwork, for the woman with ADHD, is like death by a thousand paper cuts—aka torture by tedium.

Paperwork EMS

Though many organizing books tout using the "Only Handle It Once" (OHIO) method for managing paper overflow, I find this to be unrealistic for most women with ADHD. It's helpful to use the triage approach with paperwork and focus on what is most important to deal with first. Ask yourself, *What needs to be taken care of* now?

Remember how your difficulties with executive function make decision making, sorting, and prioritizing difficult at times? That's why paperwork is so difficult for most women with ADHD, but triage can help. Let's revisit our clutter triage approach, but this time use it for papers.

Stage 1: EMS—Urgent Documents with Deadlines

Buy or select a container to hold your most important *urgent documents with deadlines*. This container will typically contain documents such as these:

- Bills: mortgage, utilities, insurance, and so on

- Renewals: driver's license, registration, and so on

- Permission slips (for kids): field trips, sports sign-ups, medication forms

Your container could be a clear plastic bin with (or without) hanging folders or a basket (wicker, cloth, metal, plastic, whatever you like). Label this container to remind you of what's in it—for example, "SOS," "URGENT," or "IMPORTANT," or whatever is meaningful for you. Store papers here that need your *immediate attention,* versus documents that are important but need long-term storage (such as your living will and durable power of attorney). The key is that the container be visible! As urgent papers come in, open each one, note the due date, and jot it down on the front of the envelope before storing it—in chronological order with the earliest due date in front—in your special file. Keep it close to where you normally handle bills and other paperwork.

If you feel like you've just won the lottery by using an SOS basket, fantastic, because you will finally have your most important documents all in one place. However, if you're really inspired to get organized and you're using a bin, you might want to use folders to break your documents down into groupings. You can label and color-code each folder— for example:

- green folder: bills with stamps and envelopes, so that you have everything handy

- yellow folder: papers needing your signature

Now you've gotten your most urgent documents handled. Let's go on to stage 2.

Stage 2: General Surgery—The Next Most Important Documents

Now find another container to store the next most important documents, ones that require some type of response from you but that are not urgent. Again, you might want to organize them into folders or just store them all together. In other words, if you don't respond to your friend's baby shower invitation, you might really hurt her feelings, but your family won't be left freezing in the dark in the middle of winter. Label this container whatever is meaningful to you, such as "NEEDS RESPONSE ASAP." This container will typically contain documents such as these that need responses but aren't critical to your health and well-being:

- party invitations

- offers to change or upgrade services

- subscription renewals

- volunteer requests

- donation requests

- appointment reminders (after you've captured them in your planner)

- school events

- maintenance service reminders (for example, for your furnace or car)

You can relax! Your most important papers are now organized by priority. But let's not forget the other papers that will still need your attention at some point down the road. That's stage 3.

Stage 3: Reconstructive Surgery—Papers for Later

This container should only hold papers that don't go in either of the first two containers. You do, however, want to review these papers at some point:

- magazines

- catalogs

- sales offerings

- public service announcements (PSAs)

- coupons/advertising booklets

- photos

- policy changes: credit cards, websites, services

- children's artwork or school projects

Label the container something that will be clear to you down the road, such as "LATER READING."

Give yourself a pat on the back, because the hardest part is over. Still, you need a system for storing important papers that you'll need to access in the future. So on we go to stage 4!

Stage 4: Post-Op—Documents for Later Access

The last container should hold items you want to keep but do not need to access in the near future or on a regular basis. This can be a filing cabinet in your basement. These may be very important documents, but they don't require any response from you:

- medical records: X-rays, reports, scans

- homeowner documents: mortgage papers, blueprints, estimates

- insurance policies: life, home, renter's, car, other

- personal letters or kids' artwork or writing (moves here from stage 3 after you've had a chance to look at it)

- pet info: medical records, care and feeding guidelines

It's best to put everything else, particularly junk mail, directly into the recycling bin.

Important: Any critical documents like stocks/bonds/mutual funds, wills, power of attorney, or life insurance policies should all go in a safe deposit box at your bank or in a fireproof lockbox.

♛

Every piece of paper you touch should go in one of these four containers. If it doesn't belong there, then pitch it!

Allow yourself, if needed, to *temporarily* store mail, magazines, catalogs, and other papers in a fifth container before sorting them into one of the four containers listed above. A decorative piece, like for example a woven basket, can make your piles of paper less visually obtrusive. This is a more realistic technique for managing papers that would otherwise be strewn on the counter and eventually lost in the heap.

When Life Gives You Papers, Make Paper Dolls (kidding!)

As much as you may want to snip into doilies or dollies every new piece of paper that passes your doorstep, that will likely create more chaos. Instead, try some of these tips to keep from getting buried alive under an avalanche of paper:

- Keep a pad of sticky notes and a pen next to every phone in your house. As calls come in or you remember something important, jot it down on a sticky note. Keep a master log for these notes in your home office or wherever you do your paperwork—a simple notebook will suffice—and never let it leave that room. Date each page of the log. At the end of each day, collect the sticky notes and affix them on the appropriate dated page in your master log. No more searching for scraps of paper, and you'll have a great system for finding important information.

- Dedicate an entire wall of your home office or wherever you do paperwork as a place to display your papers: make it half bulletin board and half whiteboard. The more you see your papers, the more likely you will be to take action.

- Instead of a small writing desk, use long tables along one end of your home office to give you plenty of space to work on your paper-related activities. Small file cabinets can be stored underneath.

- Find attractive hanging letter bins and other helpful organizers online. You can label them "Kids" or "Bills" or whatever.

- Use a buddy system to help you stay on track. Invite a friend to come over to read, knit, pay bills, write, whatever, just so that you have company while doing your most odious task.

- In your office supply area, take a sample of whatever is in a storage box and fold it over the side of the box to visually remind you what's inside.

- If you have kids:

  - Pay them to file papers for you once they are old enough.

  - Store their school papers and art projects in a large artist's portfolio and slip it under a bed. At the end of each school year, remove all pieces but one. If they are still too difficult to part with, take photos of the pieces before tossing them or save them to use as wrapping paper. Another alternative: make one large collage per school year.

  - Train them to manage their own paperwork by installing a hanging rack (like the magazine rack you see at your doctor's office) at their height on the wall in their bedrooms or possibly at their launching pads.

- Watch for tips on handling paperwork in magazines or on websites. Save the good ones—clip them out and start folders of your own, either on your computer or in store-bought binders.

For most of us, it's not easy to keep a handle on paperwork. But armed with new systems and new strategies, you will be thrilled with how much less cluttered your home and life will be. Enjoy your newfound freedom—and use some of that free time to tackle the cleaning you've been avoiding!

And There's a Reason It's Called House*work*

As wonderful as it will feel to get your papers organized, you'll also want to tackle the clutter and cleaning that need to be done elsewhere in your home. In this section, I'll share my special approach to cleaning—"laser-vision cleaning"—and some specifics for making your kitchen and home office into workable, livable spaces. But when you have to clean, where do you start?

Laser-Vision Cleaning

Difficulties with prioritizing can make it pretty hard to decide where to start cleaning. Then the feeling of being overwhelmed kicks in, which starts procrastination spinning, and before you know it, you have a veritable cascade of internal resistance. So I advocate a method I call "laser-vision cleaning": you start cleaning in one area of one room and keep going in a clockwise direction. By doing this, you don't get off track by putting things away in the next room, which then pulls you into yet another room, which then makes you feel overwhelmed or distracted like a mouse in a maze. Using your laser-vision cleaning method will help you stay with the task and keep moving until your job is done. Now let's go to the kitchen, and I'll show you how to clean it in just three steps!

Kitchen Klutter

Earlier in this chapter, we covered tips on the two top stress inducers: getting out of the house on time and dealing with paper piles. Third on our list of stress inducers from clutter and disorganization is a messy kitchen. Other than the bedroom, we spend the most time in the kitchen, which is prone to being the messiest room. We try to maintain it as well as we can, but even with our best intentions, it can easily and quickly get out of hand. Many of us are in the habit of dumping purses, mail, keys, and other junk onto the counter as soon as we enter the house. It doesn't take long for it to add up and make us crazy. So where do you start? Take the laser-vision cleaning approach (see above) and follow these three steps:

Step 1: Clear the Sink

"Emergency, emergency, no food until we clear the sink!" (sound of EMS sirens). To get anything remotely related to cooking done, washing the dishes and clearing the sink is top priority.

Step 2: Remove Unnecessary Items

Once the sink and dishes are done, you're on to general surgery. Look clockwise—no cheating—and remove any items from the counters and table that don't belong. Now this is important: *stay in the kitchen!* Arm yourself with paper or plastic bags or baskets, and when you come across mail, toys, makeup—whatever doesn't belong in the kitchen—dump it in a bag or basket. "Batch" your items—for example, items that go in your home office should go in one bag, toys go in another.

Step 3: Put Things in Their Proper Place

Once the kitchen is done, and *only* when it's done, take one bag at a time and put the items away in their proper room and space. To save yourself from running up and down the stairs, take all the upstairs batches and set them on the bottom step so you can take them all up at once.

So now your kitchen is clean and spiffy—at least the parts that you can see. But what about those cupboards? Could they use a little help, too? Here's how to organize them to make them work for *you.*

How to Organize Cupboards

To organize cupboards, pull out your old shoeboxes and give them new life as spice organizers. To make spices even easier to find, affix red sticky dots or labels on the top or side of each bottle or can and write the spice's first letter on it, along with the expiration date. Use roll-out shelves whenever possible to help store items and easily find them. Nowadays, there are even refrigerators that have these already installed. Buy lazy Susans for lower cupboards. For deep shelves, use bins for groups of foods so that they are easier to store and easier to find. For example, use one bin to store canned soups. Peel off one soup label and hang it over the edge of the bin or tape it onto the shelf underneath the bin. This way, you'll know what's back there in the dark! Go to my website, http://ADDconsults.com, for specific product names for all these things and stores where you can find them.

Now your kitchen's in good shape. Let's move on to the home office and get things in shape there.

Home Office

For those of you who work at home or simply have tons of projects, paper, and files, I highly recommend hiring a professional organizer to help you get started. Since I spend a lot of time in my home office, it was a necessity to have a professional come in, assess my space and room layout, and develop a system to keep my things organized. If that's not an option for you, consider purchasing a lot of filing cabinets—the kind that have bottoms in the drawers. I find that with open hanging filing systems, the folders often slip off the rod, spilling all the contents onto the floor. The other advantage to having bottoms is, if you have a hanging file system, you can store things under the files. If you're using an extra bedroom as your home office, add shelves in the closet and use the space for storage, or store office supplies in Pendaflex folders in your filing cabinet.

Consider utilizing online banking and online bill paying. Not only will this cut down on paper clutter, it will also make bill paying easier in general. Some businesses will even e-mail you reminders to pay your bill, an added bonus.

Bonus Tips

Now let's look at some suggestions for making general clutter management and cleaning more tolerable. These tips will help you with your chores:

- Claim your own "messy zone." This frees you up from feeling that every corner of your home must be clutter-free and perfect.

- Claim "tidy zones" in your home that must stay clean.

- Barter with family members; swap clearing clutter for some other chore you don't mind doing.

- Twin it! It can be easier to remember (and follow through) on chores when you pair two activities:

  - Clean out your kids' backpacks when helping with their homework.

  - Put away the dishes when packing lunches.

  - Empty the fridge of rotten food on garbage day.

  - When folding laundry, watch TV or listen to music (and then have a sock ball fight with the family to engage family members and have fun).

- MIF: Make it fun.

We've covered a lot of ground in finding ways to tame clutter. But in reality, most of us will still be challenged by this. How can you live with clutter and not let it damage your self-esteem?

Is Clutter Really So Bad?

If you define who you are by the amount of clutter you have in your life and become angry, depressed, or anxious as a result, then clutter has taken control of you and your self-esteem. Rather than hyperfocus on your deficits, learn to live with a bit of clutter and disorganization. It's really not the end of the world. As Dr. Ned Hallowell, ADHD expert and coauthor of the groundbreaking book *Driven to Distraction,* said in his blog (2012), "Get well enough organized to achieve your goals. The key here is 'well enough.' That doesn't mean you have to be very well organized at all—just well enough organized to achieve your goals." Let go of your idealized perfect home and focus on your strengths. You are more than your clutter!

CHAPTER 3

Newsflash! Woman Has Meltdown in Frozen Foods Aisle!

About ten years ago, I decided to have Passover dinner at my home to prove that I was, indeed, "adult" enough to entertain a houseful of guests. Passover involves about ten different dishes. Armed with all kinds of ADHD-friendly strategies, I knew exactly what I would do to make this successful with the least amount of stress. I promptly called the local catering company that specializes in holiday meals. Hah! This was going to be a slam dunk.

The big day arrived, and I picked up and put in my trunk what was close to a mortgage payment's worth of boxed food. Once home, I did another once-over to make sure the house was presentable. At 5:30 p.m., I remembered to turn on the stove. I opened up the refrigerator to pull out all the food I'd bought and stopped dead in my tracks. There was *no* food in the fridge. My mind raced. *Who took all the food? Why would someone do that?* Then it dawned on me. I'd left hundreds of dollars' worth of freshly cooked, scrumptious food in the trunk of my car in a hot garage for seven hours. Rather than change our names from Terry and Jerry to "Sam 'n' Ella," I tossed out all the food and called all my guests in a panic to cobble together the first ever Passover potluck smorgasbord.

This story is a microcosm of the types of challenges women with ADHD face. It's especially common for those who are married with children, but even single women share the expectation that they "should" be able to whip up a tasty meal for their friends now and then. Many wives and mothers, even those with partners who are supportive and willing to help, are expected to pull off dinners every night, not to mention breakfasts, lunches (including school lunches for the kids), and holiday or special occasion meals. When we falter, our self-esteem takes a real hit, and we ask ourselves, *What is wrong with me? Everyone else can get a dinner on the table effortlessly, so why can't I even decide what to make?*

Girls generally observe their mothers in the kitchen and integrate those skills into their own lives. But what if that little girl had ADHD and didn't pay attention to her mother's kitchen activities? Or what if her mother also had ADHD and struggled herself? Believe it or not, just about every aspect of food preparation requires strong executive functioning. There is the planning and shopping, which requires selecting, organizing, and choosing from literally thousands of options at the grocery store. In the kitchen, there is the multitasking and timing required to prepare a number of different foods and having them all ready at the same time. Following a recipe requires having to break tasks down into smaller steps, something most people can do without a second thought; but then up the ante by a thousand and put on full wattage pressure with the task of entertaining others, especially on a holiday, and the stress becomes completely overwhelming. This is when a woman with ADHD might end up serving up havoc instead of haddock.

The first part of this chapter outlines the most typical challenges involved in meal preparation for women with ADHD. The second part offers a myriad of solutions to help take the edge off of this daily chore.

Meal Prep: The Latest in Extreme Sports

The everyday task of meal planning is second nature to many, but for the woman with ADHD, it can take on monumental proportions. She may as well be trying to win the Tour de France in a freak snowstorm with her shoelaces tied together—every day. Most people don't recognize all the basic tasks that go into meal preparation, many of which require healthy executive functioning:

- meal planning
- grocery shopping
- food storage
- cooking
- cleanup

Let's "unpack" each one of these steps to see what's inside.

Meal Planning Is for Sissies

Most women with ADHD will tell you that meal planning is great in theory. Most will also tell you that they have no clue what they're serving until 5:00 p.m., and then they are scrambling to throw something together—like scrambled eggs! Or the old standby, cereal and milk, if they're lucky enough to have a carton of milk that isn't curdled. Meal planning seems like such a no-brainer, right? Not to the brain with ADHD.

Why is meal planning like juggling twelve balls while roller skating? Because people with ADHD have difficulties with the executive functioning and working memory areas of the brain. In the online factsheet "The Important Role of Executive Functioning and Self-Regulation in ADHD," Dr. Russell Barkley (2011, used with permission), leading ADHD researcher and expert, explains executive functioning as "those neuropsychological processes needed to sustain problem solving toward a goal." Working memory, the ability to hold information in your mind for a few minutes to a few hours, is the foundation of executive functioning; it allows you to plan ahead, organize, pay attention, and problem-solve. Meal planning involves going from step 1 to step 2 and then from step 2 to step 3 without getting distracted and ultimately getting thrown off course.

Sensory Overload in the Grocery Aisle

Many women with ADHD are hypersensitive to stimuli. This can make a trip to the local supermarket feel like being in the middle of Times Square on New Year's Eve. For example, have you ever walked into a supermarket and felt like you were going to have a seizure? Perhaps your head started spinning when you saw ten thousand colorful package labels row after row on shelves, screaming, "Pick me! Pick me!" You found yourself singing along with the Muzak, losing track of what to do next. The horrific fluorescent lighting made you feel a tad seasick. The sound of screaming babies and whiny young children bored through your brain with the intensity of a lightning bolt. The smell of household cleaners flowed into the deli, and you felt sickened by the competing scents. The whole experience of grocery shopping may be so overwhelming that you avoid it as much as possible—until you're down to your last roll of toilet paper. So buying the food is hard enough, but that's just the beginning. Once you get home, you have to put away the groceries. No problem, right? Wrong!

Seven Bottles of Ketchup and No Milk

How many times have you searched for a crucial ingredient in your kitchen only to shut down because your cabinets, cupboards, and pantry are so disorganized that you can't find what you need? It's the old seven-bottles-of-ketchup-but-no-milk syndrome.

Though desperate to have a system, you usually *don't* have one, and if you do, it's generally short-lived. Coming home from the grocery store, food is often haphazardly put away because it simply takes too much mental and physical effort, especially after hours of sensory assault at the market, to keep up an organized system. You may as well be blind when putting away the groceries. Even under the best of circumstances, it's almost impossible to set up a system because of your difficulty seeing the big picture. Further, spatial relationships create quite the challenge: how do you fit all those frozen foods into that small freezer? It's like playing a game of Tetris, manipulating packages so that everything fits in neatly. Not an easy task for a woman with ADHD.

There's a neurologically based "out of sight, out of mind" mind-set for women with ADHD. This results in a lot of duplications and waste because you've forgotten about those seven bottles of ketchup sitting way in the back of the cupboard or that now-rotting second big bag of pre-washed salad mix shoved into the back of the fridge.

How Cooking Can Leave You Boiling with Rage, Half-Baked, or Just Plain Raw

It seems that most women have a flair for multitasking, and though some women with ADHD often *do* multitask well in certain situations, cooking is often not one of them. Think about it. Cooking requires all of these brain functions:

- transitioning

- multitasking

- staying focused (dealing with distractions)

- timing

- paying attention to detail

Let's take a closer look at each of these functions. Below are some examples of real-life challenges that can be roadblocks to seamless, successful food prep.

Transitioning

For many (but not all) women with ADHD, it's more enjoyable to do just about anything *but* cook. We know that the ADHD brain craves stimulation. For the woman with ADHD, spending time online, watching TV, gardening, or engaging in other stimulating activities are much more satisfying than something as banal as meal planning. These types of pleasurable activities can capture one's attention for hours on end. So, though many think of ADHD as an *inability* to pay attention, it's actually the inability to consistently *sustain* attention, especially with boring tasks.

Transitioning out of a pleasurable activity and into a boring or frustrating one borders on the impossible, so naturally procrastination and avoidance kick in. In fact, transitioning from one activity to another is often difficult in general for women with ADHD. Nancy Ratey, EdM (2010), internationally recognized authority on ADHD coaching, writes as a guest blogger for Children and Adults with ADHD (CHADD)'s ADHD Coach blog, "Transitions require the brain to shift its focus and attention. The ADHD brain often overreacts to this discontinuity by going into a 'startle' state, making the person anxious and stressed." Is this how you feel in the kitchen?

Multitasking

You're stirring the pot of pasta while keeping an eye on the chicken in the oven. The oven timer goes off, but you forgot to start slicing tomatoes for the salad. You end up leaving the chicken in too long because you're back tending the pasta. You pull the chicken out of the oven and drain the pasta so that the chicken doesn't get cold. You forget to cut up the lettuce that's been sitting in the fridge and end up throwing the tomatoes on a plate. Again, dinner is overcooked chicken, undercooked pasta, and no green vegetable.

The example above demonstrates executive functioning gone wrong. Think of executive functioning as the orchestra conductor of the brain, who coordinates planning, organizing, paying attention, and following steps. When there is executive dysfunction, confusion and disorganization occur, much like what would happen in an orchestra if the conductor was blindfolded and wearing earplugs.

Staying Focused

You're already looking for any excuse to get out of the boring job of meal prep, so when you remember that there was a story you wanted to catch on the 6:00 p.m. news, you promise yourself you'll only leave the kitchen for five minutes. But, oh, my god, the story is *fascinating*! While in the family room, you notice the pile of newspapers and toss them into the recycle bin in the garage. While in the garage, you decide to take the garbage to the curb. While outside, you notice some flowers wilting and decide to pick, oh, just a few dying petals off. Twenty-five minutes later when you're back in the kitchen, the rice is scorched, ruining your pot and your dinner and leaving the "lovely" scent of charred rice in the air. You sit down on the kitchen floor and want to cry.

People with ADHD find it very difficult to stick to a single task when there are other competing stimuli, whether it's hearing the sound of a radio, seeing something interesting out of the corner of their eye, or thinking of an upcoming vacation. Simply put, people with ADHD have difficulties blocking out distractions. Scientists believe this is due to differences in neurobiological chemicals in the brain, such as dopamine.

Timing

Anyone who cooks a lot can tell you that putting on a great meal has everything to do with timing. People with ADHD are notoriously challenged when it comes to time management and a sense of time in general. An hour can feel like a minute to them, and a minute can feel like an hour. Though it may seem that the food has been cooking for ten minutes, in reality, that ten minutes can easily slip into forty-five. There goes another meal burned to a crisp.

Trying to get everything ready and placed on the table at the same time can feel like being the ringmaster of a three-ring circus: chicken takes an hour in the oven, rice boils for twenty minutes, peas for five.

And if you're brave enough to add sauce for a bit of pizzazz, that's another step to figure out. It's much easier to pick up the phone and call 1-800-SEND-DINNER.

Paying Attention to Detail: Tedium Is the Enemy

Since meal planning is such a chore for the woman with ADHD, she is often reduced to repetition to help simplify things. But then she has to contend with boredom of preparing the same meals week in and week out. Yawn!

As previously mentioned, people with ADHD thrive on stimuli. Brain scans show that when people with ADHD are forced to do boring tasks, the prefrontal cortex slows down, causing sluggishness. In order to be productive, focused, and alert, the ADHD brain needs a higher level of stimulation than the non-ADHD brain.

Add repetitive chopping and measuring to that, and, oh, my! For women with ADHD, paying attention to details and doing math are often areas of challenge—and recipes call for both. What sort of pan is used for omelets? Which rack is the middle rack? How high is a high temperature? How many teaspoons are in a tablespoon? How does one cut a recipe in half? (That said, note that though these examples are targeted toward women who would rather do anything *but* be in the kitchen, some women with ADHD are, in fact, exceptional cooks and find cooking to be a stimulating, creative experience—everything but the cleanup, that is. More on cleanup in a moment.)

Juggling the Family's Needs

There are plenty of challenges in the kitchen when the house is empty, but if you have a family and are trying to cook when the family is home, all hell breaks loose. The kids and hubby are eager to share their day with you, and there's lots of bustle, with people ducking in and out of the kitchen, throwing you off course faster than a ship without a compass. It's also the time of day when irritability strikes. Everyone is tired and hungry. If you're the primary chef of the house, or it's your night to cook and your meal is running late, or someone is unhappy with the choice you made for dinner, or if you are feeling stressed, any one of you might just get *hangry* (hungry + angry = hangry). And that's when things can get ugly.

The Grand Finale: Cleanup

If you have a partner and your partner handles the cleanup (or better yet, cooking *and* cleanup), lucky for you; but if that's not the case, then you're on to the grand finale of the meal. After a full day's work, you've struggled through planning, shopping, prepping, and cooking, and then the end of the day arrives: cleanup. Why is that such an ordeal? By the time you've prepared the meal, you are so wiped out, the thought of clearing the table, let alone washing dishes, is about as appealing as climbing Mount Everest. And if you work outside the home, your more important job is waiting for you: being a partner/spouse and/or mom. So typically the dirty dishes either sit where they were last touched by human hands or are dumped in the sink for later attention. This, of course, means waking up to a huge mess the next morning—not a great way to start the day. Again, the issue of boredom gets in the way. Who wants to stand there washing and drying, or even loading the dishwasher, when there are much more interesting or relaxing things to do before retiring for the night?

Entertaining: Don't Call Me, I'll Call You

Entertaining. Ugh. Now you're doing all the things you normally struggle with, but you're also doing it "on stage." It's like the fear of cooking on steroids. Women with ADHD typically already feel inadequate in so many areas and try to hide their perceived shortcomings. Putting on a bash can accentuate these feelings of shame and not being able to measure up. After all, it's one thing to serve your family mac 'n' cheese because you forgot to pick up the buns that were to go with the hamburgers. It's another thing to forget to buy ten steaks for the four couples who will arrive at your home in an hour. There is the additional stress of planning for any guests who have food sensitivities, food allergies, dietary restrictions, or particular preferences because they are vegetarians, nondrinkers, and so on. Then there's the added pressure of making sure the house is presentable. That alone could give any woman with ADHD a reason *not* to open her home to guests!

Tips for Surviving Kitchen Duty

Now that we know how meal planning, shopping, cooking, and entertaining are often areas of deficit and difficulty for women with ADHD, let's explore the many tips and suggestions that will make life in the kitchen more manageable. The solutions below include food prep shortcuts, tips for avoiding sensory overload when shopping, visual cues, and other strategies that can go a long way to take the stress out of meal preparation and restore the pleasure of spending quality time with your family or friends around the table.

Meal Planning for Single or Group Servings

Utilizing organizing techniques for the kitchen is imperative for helping you to survive while cooking in it. Here are some questions to ask yourself:

- Are you more comfortable following recipes, or are you more of an easygoing, creative cook?

- How do you come up with recipe ideas?

- How do you decide which days to serve which meals?

- How do you plan your meals and shop for the ingredients?

If you are single:

- How do you shop for one person to avoid wasting food due to spoilage?

- Where can you find simple, easy to prepare, tasty meal ideas for one?

- How best can you store fresh or prepared food for single servings?

If you have a family:

- How do you take into account all your family members' needs, such as food preferences, allergies, time restrictions, and so on?

- If your children have after-school activities, how do you fit in meal planning and cooking on those nights?

- If you're running late from work, what plans do you have in place for getting dinner on the table?

In order to address these questions, it's helpful to have strategies to keep you on task. You can jot down meal ideas in your planner so you're not rushing at the last minute to put something on the table. This includes choosing your shopping days. Your smartphone is also a fantastic tool for keeping track of what ingredients and supplies are needed. There are tons of apps that can also suggest meals according to what ingredients you happen to already have at hand. Use online recipe websites or quick and easy cookbooks to come up with additional ideas, especially for those days when you're rushing and need some shortcut meals.

Plan or Starve (POS) Method

Using visual cues and tangible reminders comes in handy when striving to remember chores and routines. My POS method is a unique way to make meal planning and grocery shopping less stressful. Here's how it works:

1. Gather enough index cards to cover seven to ten dinner menus, one menu per card.

2. On each card, write out the entire meal for one night—for example, roast chicken, mashed potatoes, and green beans. If a

recipe is needed, write down the name of the cookbook and the page number.

3. Write down the approximate amount of time needed to prepare and cook the meal.

4. On the other side of the card, list all the ingredients needed.

5. If it's a quick and easy recipe requiring less than 15 minutes of prep, make a notation like a red star or "QE" (quick and easy).

6. Look at your planner first thing in the morning. (Use of a planner will be addressed in chapter 4, on time management.) Choose a card that matches your schedule for the day/evening.

Having this system in place automatically removes the worry about deciding *what* to make. Use your QE cards for those nights you're working late or rushing kids to late afternoon sports practices, music classes, or other activities. Keep the cards in the kitchen for quick reference. To see a short video of what my POS meal plan looks like and how the system works, visit http://youtu.be/-Y-ik3Z5CDY.

Some women have a system of making the same thing every week—for example, chicken on Monday, spaghetti on Tuesday—and rotating. Others need a list visible at all times, reminding them what to make for dinner that night. They take that list to the store each day and buy the needed ingredients.

Grocery Shopping Anti-Stressors

You can never have too many tricks in your back pocket when it comes to making shopping an easier task. Below are a few tips to help reduce the stress of grocery shopping:

• To avoid sensory overload when grocery shopping, shop at smaller, quieter markets.

• To avoid the tendency to overshop, bring a shopping list or take along your POS cards.

- To avoid feeling overwhelmed by the chaos of a lot of people, shop at off times.

- Wear a headset and listen to calming music.

- Leave the kids at home.

- For larger stores, draw a diagram so you know exactly where to go to find your items.

Now that you have some strategies up your sleeve, you can delete the local pizzeria's phone number from your speed dial. Below are some kitchen tips to help with meal prep.

Shortcuts in the Kitchen

If you hate cooking as much as I do, you'll want to gather as many ideas as possible to make this task easier on you. Here are some tips to lighten your load:

- Use bagged salads (just toss in precooked chicken strips for a complete meal).

- Use frozen items for side dishes, such as vegetable medleys, pasta, rolls, and so on.

- Have breakfast for dinner. It's quick and easy to make scrambled eggs with traditional sides.

- Make double recipes and freeze the leftovers for a later date.

- Keep baggies of cooked ground beef in the freezer for sloppy joes, tacos, or spaghetti dinners.

People who enjoy cooking often have lots of shortcuts. If you have friends who like to cook, ask them about some of their favorite shortcuts.

Bonus Tips

Planning meals for a family is always a challenge. If you need a little help on that front, here are a few more tips:

- Have a second set of POS cards written up and stored in your purse so you can reference them at the grocery store. No more forgetting ingredients!

- Laminate the cards for longevity.

- Picky eaters at home? Let your children take turns pulling a card from the stack. They'll be more willing to eat what you make if they have a choice in the matter.

- Brainstorm menu ideas with your family. The more you involve the kids, the more likely they will eat what you've prepared.

There is nothing wrong with bringing in dinner two, three, even five times a week if it's within your budget. Says Sheila, a woman I worked with years back:

My husband was always on a diet, and my two kids had not a single meal they liked in common other than take-out pizza. One ate chicken; the other hated it. One loved pasta; the other gagged on it. Cooking was difficult for me, but the idea of making two to three different meals every night put me over the edge. Though the pediatrician told me not to give in, I just couldn't see one or the other child eat cereal every night, so I threw in the towel and picked up meals everyone would enjoy. I fit it into my budget by removing luxuries like cable TV. To me, carryout was not a luxury. It was a necessity.

Eating out frequently is also an option if your budget can handle it. This solves the problem of choosing meals that please everyone in the family. Children especially seem to enjoy buffet- or cafeteria-style restaurants.

Others have found success in bartering. If your spouse or teenager enjoys cooking, swap out cooking for cleaning up or something else that he or she hates to do. Some people even barter with friends. Consider babysitting or gardening for a friend or relative in exchange for a week's worth of prepared meals.

In many towns, there are "chop shops" where you can put together an entire week's worth of meals in just a couple hours by using their prepped food, tools, recipes, and containers. Then you can just pop them in the freezer when you get home. Go with a friend or your kids for a fun outing.

Since meal prep can be hazardous to some women's self-esteem, I consider these shortcuts and strategies to be accommodations, much like the special support a child who is struggling in school needs in order to be successful. There is no shame in getting the help you need.

Food Storage Tips

You can never have too many tips to help you with organizing your kitchen. Below are a few more ideas for organizing and storing your food items:

- Next time you're in the market for a new fridge, buy the largest one possible within your budget. You'll be able to see items better instead of having to search behind jars and bottles for what you need.

- For pantry and cabinets, install shelves that roll out. No more searching in the black pit.

- Purchase clear plastic containers, fill them up with your staple foods, and label them. Organize your space by placing items used most frequently in front and by category, such as cereals, canned soup, and so on.

- Draw diagrams of the inside of the pantry and cabinets so that it's easier to remember where to store items. Tape the diagram to the inside of the door.

It may take some time to make these changes in your kitchen, but it will be time well spent. Being able to see where your food is or where it should be stored will in the long run save you not only time but also a lot of frustration.

Bonus Tips

Below are some extra tips to keep your momentum going. Use these as starters; I'm sure you'll come up with more once you get rolling.

- Keep a shopping list taped to the inside of your pantry and other food storage areas. When you're down to your last box of pasta, for example, write down "pasta" on your list.

- Use a preprinted shopping list with check boxes so you can check off items that you need.

- Show family members where the shopping list is. If they finish the last carton of milk, they write "milk" on the list.

- Make your own preprinted shopping list on your computer. Include staples that you buy frequently, and leave blank lines for items you don't buy as often.

You've asked friends and relatives for cooking shortcuts. The Internet has hundreds of websites with food storage tips, too, so take advantage of those resources.

Whiz-Bang Cooking

Whether you're a whiz in the kitchen (and I don't mean Cheez Whiz), or you bump and bang your way through meal prep, you can benefit from these snappy shortcuts. Sticky notes, index card reminders, timers, even mini posters with step-by-step instructions are all helpful aids for getting through meal preparation.

It's okay to use shortcuts, such as premixed, prepared meals, but do your best to avoid buying foods with lots of preservatives and added chemicals. Shopping at discount wholesale stores that don't allow additives or preservatives in their foods will not only save you money but also guarantee that all the food you purchase is free of chemical additives. Go to my website, http://ADDconsults.com, for specific product names and stores. It can also be useful to keep lots of healthy snacks around the house—such as foods with protein, like yogurt and cheese—as these seem to help ADHD brains with attention and calming. Using recipes with fewer than five steps and fewer than five ingredients is ideal. In fact, feel free to toss out or donate all those cookbooks sitting around gathering dust. If you haven't used them in two years, ditch them.

Know your own biological temperament. If you're a morning person, prep dinner when you are finished with breakfast. If you're a night owl, experiment with using a crockpot and throwing all the ingredients in the night before. Then stick the pot in the fridge until morning when you can turn it on and come home to a ready-made hot dinner.

It's never too early to engage the kids. Even a five-year-old can set a table or help with prep and cleanup.

If you're lucky and have the budget, hire someone to prepare your meals. There's no need to feel guilty! You are making an accommodation for your ADHD brain.

Tips for Cleanup

You're not the only one who hates kitchen cleanup! Below are a few more tips to help get done what you *really* don't want to do:

- Stop being the martyr. If you're cooking, have the family clean up. Take turns.

- Wash the dishes as you go so that you're not overwhelmed with a pile of pots and pans after dinner. Tell yourself you're rewarding yourself with a clean kitchen after your meal so that you'll be free to relax and not have to think about a messy kitchen.

- Have a transition signal. Tell yourself that in order to watch TV, you *must* first clean up the kitchen.

- Visualize a clean kitchen and remind yourself how good it will feel when you wake up in the morning and enter that tidy kitchen rather than a messy one.

- Make a bargain with yourself: clean up half the kitchen mess after dinner and half in the morning. For example, load and run the dishwasher after dinner, but unload and put away dishes in the morning.

If you find it helpful, offer yourself a reward for completing the cleanup. It could be a relaxing bath, some computer time, or a fun game with your kids. Just make it something you'll enjoy.

Tips for Entertaining

You might just surprise yourself and find that, with these tools, you want to entertain more often. Who knows? Maybe you'll be the next Martha Stewart. Okay, maybe not...but do use these tips to help reduce the stress of entertaining:

- If you hate it, don't do it!

- Go out when you meet with friends instead of having people over to the house.

- Consider having a potluck in the backyard or bring in pizza for an informal, fun get-together. There are no rules that say you must cook the entire meal or have formal seating in the house. The idea is to connect with people, not showcase your culinary talents (or lack thereof).

- Be your authentic self. If others invite you to their house, and you feel you can't reciprocate, invite them to go out to dinner as your guests. Stop trying to keep up with the Joneses.

- If your spouse loves to cook and entertain, hand the duty over with a smile. Perhaps you could swap cooking for cleanup or some other household chore.

- Instead of having an entire dinner, invite friends over for dips or desserts and drinks.

- Having a holiday freak-out? What's wrong with heading to the restaurant for Thanksgiving dinner? Or have it at someone else's house and offer to bring one thing that you feel comfortable handling. When my mother hosted holiday dinners, she knew to only ask me to bring the relish tray. Or you can offer to pay your friends or relatives for the food in exchange for use of their home and preparation.

As my parents began aging and found it difficult to cook and host holiday dinners, I offered to bring them fully cooked, prepared carryout meals. Even so, it was hard for me to gauge how to reheat things or which containers to use, how to time the heat-up, and which things to put in the oven first. Even carryout can be a challenge when it's for a large gang, especially if you're not that familiar with the kitchen!

Meal planning, cooking, cleaning up, and entertaining are not typically areas of strength for most women with ADHD, though there are the shining exceptions. But girls are often raised with the societal expectation of becoming the nurturing parent, so offering daily, nutritious meals gulped down by an appreciative family is something many women strive for. It's a symbol of love and connection with our families. But when a seemingly easy task feels unreachable, self-esteem plummets. Hopefully, you will come to a point of self-acceptance where you don't feel valued by how many bites of healthy, delicious home-cooked food your family consumes; instead, you'll come to celebrate time with your family, partner, or yourself as the priority, even if it means dinner comes in a plastic container. It's time for you to make the rules in the kitchen. Hopefully, all the tips in this chapter will help you get back on track.

CHAPTER 4

Tick-Tock…Trouble!

"I'm so sorry—I know I'm late," said Liz to Donna, the receptionist at her dentist's office, "but I was trying to find a parking space when I realized that I had left all my change at home, so I parked illegally just for a minute to run into a store to buy a pack of gum to get change for the meter, but the line was really long, and there was a fascinating article in *Newsweek* at the checkout counter, and by the time I got back, my car had been towed and then…" Liz saw the frown forming on Donna's face.

"Liz, this is the third time in a row that you've been late," said Donna.

"Oh, I know, I know, I screwed up again, didn't I? I'm soooo sorry! But I'm only, like what…thirty minutes late?"

"Your appointment was an hour ago, and we can't keep everyone else waiting. That's not fair. My next opening isn't for another month," Donna said with a long sigh.

Liz melted into the floor with shame. She felt as if she were back twenty years, hearing her seventh-grade math teacher, Mrs. Kravitch, chastise her again.

Running, Running, I'm So Tired of Running…Late

This kind of scenario may happen to the average person once, maybe twice in a lifetime, but for women with ADHD, it happens a lot! Hyperfocusing, distraction, and forgetfulness happen throughout the course of every day. Women with ADHD are often overwhelmed, partly because of the ADHD, but also because, as women, they are trying to take care of everyone else around them. Being overwhelmed can lead to procrastination, which often leads to being chronically late for deadlines and appointments. Being chronically late can take a toll on your self-esteem and damage your relationships. You've probably heard your whole life that you are uncaring, selfish, immature, or worse. Executive function impairment is tied directly to a distorted sense of time and a struggle to manage it. One of the top specialists in the field of research on ADHD, Dr. Russell Barkley (2011, 2) states that "time and the future are the enemies of people with EF [executive function] difficulties when it comes to task accomplishment or performance toward a goal." It can be a daily struggle to get to places on time or to finish projects by the deadline. But executive function isn't the only part of the brain that interferes with effective time management. Short-term memory issues also have a role to play.

When Your "Working" Memory Isn't Working

A shortage of working memory (also known as short-term storage) is often troublesome for women with ADHD. In her book *Improving Working Memory: Supporting Students' Learning*, Dr. Tracy Packiam Alloway (2010, 1) describes it simply and adequately when she says, "The best way to think of working memory is as the brain's 'Post-it note.'" In other words, working memory is a short-term "holding area" for retaining a phone number you just heard, for example, or remembering the name of a person whom you've just met. In an article, Melissa Healy (2009, 1) of the *LA Times* quotes Dr. Eric Saslow, a UCLA pediatric neurologist who works with patients with cognitive deficits and learning disabilities: "Time awareness has to be connected with being able to retain in one's mind the things that are in progress and upcoming—and right there is the connection to working memory." Thus, you end up late to work *again* because you forgot to grab your purse on the way out the door.

What Results from These Cognitive Challenges?

If your working memory and executive function are impaired, then it will be extremely difficult to have an internal sense of time that cues you on getting to places on time and judging how long it takes to complete a task. (You're more likely to under- or overestimate the time needed). These contribute to the likelihood that you will be chronically late, procrastinate on important projects, avoid unpleasant tasks, and simply forget to do things. Time seems to simply fly out the window.

Help, My Clock Is Melting!!!

Do you remember as a student being bored to tears when presented with subjects that didn't hold your attention? Perhaps civics class felt like three hours instead of forty-five minutes. This concept of distorted time is perfectly illustrated in Salvador Dali's famous painting *The Persistence of Memory*, which depicts a group of melting clocks dripping like ice cream in the hot sun. Here's what happens with your sense of time:

- It moves too slowly if you're bored.

- It moves too quickly if you're mentally stimulated and involved in pleasurable activities.

- Time is either "now" or "not now" because of a fuzzy sense of past and future.

Your time distortions can also lead to procrastination. This is one of the most common and debilitating ADHD-related behaviors.

Dilly, Dally, Dawdle, and the Big Bad Wolf of Procrastination

Lots of people procrastinate, especially when it comes to dreaded chores like paying taxes or tackling overwhelming household projects like cleaning an entire basement. But as a woman with ADHD, you're likely to procrastinate on a daily basis when facing seemingly simple tasks like emptying a dishwasher or returning a phone call. It is understandable to put off such chores if, for you, a ten-minute task feels like a three-hour chore. Here are some reasons *why* you tend to procrastinate:

- You fear failure or success.

- You want everything to be perfect (perfectionism).

- You feel overwhelmed by big goals.

- You find a task unpleasant or boring.

- You fear that it will take too long to complete a task.

Unfortunately, there's a huge price to pay for your procrastination. Not only do things remain undone, but it takes a toll on your mental and physical well-being.

My Brain Works Better Under Pressure, but My Body Doesn't

When we've procrastinated on a project until the deadline looms, our adrenaline kicks in and gets us moving at the last minute. We may meet the deadline, but the work probably isn't our best. Chronic procrastination can have other negative outcomes as well:

- loss of sleep—staying up late or not sleeping because of anxiety due to the consequences of not starting or finishing a project

- health issues due to stress

- feelings of shame about not being able to get things done

- lowering of your standards just because you've run out of time, even though you know you're capable of doing better

When procrastinating, you *know* you need to get something done. But what about *forgetting* to get things done?

Did I Forget to Meet You at 4:00 p.m.?
I Can't Remember!

Holy cow! You've been looking forward to this forever. You scored two great seats to see James Taylor, your musical idol, with your best friend. The night of the concert, you're out to dinner with your mother when you get a call from your friend at the concert hall, wondering where you are. You can't just dump your mom to get to the concert. Another great outing ruined because your impaired working memory caused you to forget to check your planner for that night's schedule. Though there are lots of reasons why you may run late, procrastinate, or forget, there are also just as many tricks, tools, and technologies to help you keep track of time.

Taking the "Sting" Out of
Time Management

Though this may all sound like doom and gloom up until now, take heart! You *can* move beyond your time distortion, procrastination, and forgetfulness by utilizing some or all of the tips and tools below.

Dr. Russell Barkley explains in his book *ADHD and the Nature of Self-Control* (1997, 335) that people with ADHD need frequent external reminders and cues because their internal guides are less effective: "ADHD is more a problem of doing what one knows rather than of knowing what to do." It's not that you don't know how to do things; it's being able to do what you already know by using some simple strategies to help you stay the course.

Know Thyself: How to Track Your Time

First, let's focus on how to track and prioritize your time. Below are some strategies to help raise your awareness of how you spend your time and how effective your time management is. Don't let this scare you! It will only take you minutes to do, but it'll save you many, many hours of agony.

♕

Typical Day Assessment

By completing this little exercise, you'll have a better under-standing of how you spend your time. Take a few minutes to fill in this chart or create one of your own. Recall a typical day (the more recent, the better) and include both personal and work time on it. Break it down as far as you can into increments no smaller than fifteen minutes. Be honest, as no one will see this but you. Assign each activity a letter indicating its importance: A, B, or C. After completion, consider whether or not you are making the best possible use of the time that you have by record-ing a few observations. See the examples at the top of the chart that follows to give you an idea of how to complete it.

Time (minutes—no less than 15)	Activity (general description)	Importance (A, B, or C)	Observation (Thoughts? Feelings?)
Example: 8–10 a.m. (2 hours)	Did two loads of laundry	B	Took less time than I expected
Example: 10 – 10:15 a.m. (15 minutes)	Vacuumed family room and living room	C	Realized I can do this while doing laundry = happy! Time saver!

With ADHD, it's common to see lots of time being spent on activities of low importance. But this is the first step in becoming aware of just how you spend your day, and awareness leads to change, so you're already making good progress!

♛

Taking the "Guess" Out of Estimating Time

If you're always late leaving the gate, perhaps it's because you've never really figured out just how long it takes to do all of your daily activities. Often, people with ADHD focus on what time they need to *arrive* at work, appointments, or school, but they don't take into account hidden time eaters like traffic or even spending time searching for their keys. Here are some tips to help with estimating your "real" time:

Focus on what time you need to *leave*: Think of what time you need to leave the house instead of the time you need to arrive at your destination. Take into account all the things that can—and will—throw you off track time-wise, and build those into your departure time.

Add additional time: Here's a rule of thumb—add fifteen to thirty minutes to every routine departure time, because it's almost a given that something will throw you off course. Even avoiding things like bill paying can be resolved once you figure out how long, on average, it takes to get this done. For example, you may put off paying your bills each month because it seems like it takes forever. Next time, set a timer to see just how long it actually takes. You'll undoubtedly be surprised that it is far less than you thought. Or perhaps it takes longer because you didn't factor in gathering supplies such as envelopes, stamps, or pens. Next time, add in an extra thirty minutes for preparation, including a possible run to the office supplies store.

Time yourself: Time yourself and document how long it actually takes to complete a specific task or chore. This helps to make the subjective objective. You'll now have a factual measurement for future reference. Be sure to include "invisible time eaters" like gathering your stuff before leaving the house (for example, purse, keys, and phone), walking from your car to your destination, grabbing the newspaper, or stopping for gas.

There are many, many tasks that you do each day. Consider these typical daily routines when doing your estimates:

- getting ready in the morning (from the moment the alarm goes off to getting out the door)

- making breakfast

- packing your and/or your kids' lunches

- getting to work (from the time you leave the house to the time you sit down in your office)

- driving your kids to school

- making dinner

- tidying up the house

Once you've seen in black and white just how long such things take, you might be amazed that many of them take less time than you thought. Knowing this, you may be less inclined to procrastinate. Now, let's look at how to better manage your day.

Practice Planning and Prioritizing

Prioritizing is another hurdle for those with poor executive functioning. If you can't figure out what you need to do first, second, third, and so on, everything begins to get jumbled, and before you know it, your brain is running in circles. Even with your best intentions, your day becomes unproductive and you become anxious, stressed, and maybe even depressed.

The Almighty Planner

The creative, free-floating ADHD brain often has a love/hate relationship with a planner. You need consistency and a prioritized list to get things done, yet you hate the confines of living your day via a bulleted list. However, since you're most likely a disorganized, procrastinating type, it's imperative to use some sort of system to keep you on target. So bite the bullet and use a planner. Here are some tips:

- A simple notebook is fine. Your planner doesn't have to be fancy. Use whatever works for you.

- Purchase a planner with quarter-hour segments to help break down your day and projects into doable parts to help keep you from being overwhelmed.

- Use newer technology planners, such as those found on a smartphone or your computer. There are tons of to-do list apps for smartphones. And most smartphones have a note function built in that you can use for your to-do list.

- If you're a stay-at-home mom, treat it like any other job and get that planner! You will be amazed at how much structure it can bring to an otherwise chaotic day full of interruptions.

- Set aside time every day to plan your day. Morning people, plan your day early in the morning. Night owls, plan for the following day the evening before.

The Time-Honored To-Do List

If you prefer a paper-based system, learn to use a to-do list. Again, everyone has her own preferences, but here are some ideas that you might find helpful:

1. Date your to-do list.

2. Write out your to-do list items.

3. Prioritize your list by marking each item A, B, or C, in order of importance:

   - A = must do today, very important
   - B = need to do but not necessarily today
   - C = can wait until you have free time

4. Place a number next to each item according to urgency within a lettered group. Ask, "How time sensitive is it?" Number 1 is most important. So the letters indicate importance, but the numbers indicate both urgency *and* sequence.

5. If you find there are too many items on your list, subtract or swap some to prevent being overwhelmed.

6. Use your list!

Are you still not quite sure where to start? Let's walk through a sample to-do list to help make the process a bit clearer.

Sample To-Do List

Date your list—for example, December 1.
Make list:

- grocery shopping

- call Mom

- call Clara

- file work papers

- make travel arrangements for trip to Canada

- go to doctor appointment

- pick up birthday card for Elena

- send birthday card to Elena

- start dinner

Now, rank by importance and urgency using letters. (Hint: "A" ratings often include appointments and/or promises or commitments you've made to someone, but it depends on the nature of the commitment.)

- A: grocery shopping

- A: call Mom

- B: call Clara

- C: file work papers

- B: make travel arrangements for trip to Canada

- A: go to doctor appointment

- B: pick up birthday card for Elena

- C: send birthday card to Elena

- A: start dinner

Now, do *another* level of prioritizing within each group of lettered items. Rank each item in the letter group by importance and sequence using numbers. You may want to reorder them after ranking them to make things even clearer, as shown:

- A-1: grocery shopping

- A-2: call Mom

- A-3: go to doctor appointment

- A-4: start dinner

- B-1: make travel arrangements for trip to Canada

- B-2: pick up birthday card for Elena

- B-3: call Clara

- C-1: send birthday card to Elena

- C-2: file work papers

This helps you identify and prioritize all of your A tasks. At the end of the day, even if you don't get any of the B or C items done, you will have completed the most important tasks of the day. Here are some additional tips:

- Make all your phone calls at the same time, or "batch" them by a set schedule. Let the answering machine take a message while you're working. That's what it's for!

- Color-code tasks by priority using highlighters: red = urgent, green = should do, blue = can wait.

- Note tasks by time of day (that is, when they should be done) by marking "a.m." or "p.m." in the margin.

- Get a vibrating watch alarm. Set it to go off every thirty minutes. Check in with yourself to see if you're doing what you should be doing or if you've gone off task. See http://ADDconsults.com for a watch that vibrates, which you can also program to display customized messages, making it a great tool to remind yourself when, say, to take your meds.

- Use alarms on your computer or smartphone.

- Check out the many apps available for time management and/ or to-do lists.

- Use a whiteboard with different colored markers to remind you what is important and urgent. Red could be DO NOW. Blue could be LATER THIS WEEK. Black could be long-term projects that aren't urgent.

- Use a visual "parking lot" for brilliant ideas you don't want to lose track of. Use another whiteboard, a spiral notebook, a pack of sticky notes stored in a decorative bowl, an empty tissue box, or a bulletin board. Don't underestimate the value of your parking lot. It's a way to honor the creative impulse and remember your ideas, but it also helps you not get pulled away from your task at hand.

- Use three boards: one for current, important projects; one for less important projects; and one for your parking lot.

Learning new skills can be daunting, but stick with it. Ultimately, they will make your life easier. Now that you have some tools under your belt to help you prioritize your time, let's dive into some specific tips on avoiding procrastination.

Flipping the "Off" Switch on Procrastination

It's helpful to look within to better understand how your brain wiring contributes to procrastination, which in turn affects your productivity. The tips below will help you move forward while recognizing and acknowledging your underlying ADHD neurobiology:

Listen to your gut: Just as you did with addressing clutter, prioritize your day by simply asking how you're feeling and how much better you'd feel if you got a specific task done. What would make you feel like a million bucks if you could cross it off your to-do list? Get the most important tasks done and out of the way, and you'll free up more energy to take on other tasks. When I'm spinning, not knowing what to do first, I feel it in my stomach. You may feel it in your shoulders or experience headaches. It's important to listen to these symptoms of stress.

Work at your peak time: It also helps to take on more difficult projects or tasks during the time of the day that you have the most energy. For example, if you're a morning person, you might plow through the more mentally or physically challenging projects early in the day when you're at your performance peak.

Time on/time off: Since maintaining consistent mental effort (like writing reports, for example) for sustained periods of time can often be difficult for people with ADHD, work in short spurts: fifteen minutes on/ fifteen minutes off. If you tend to wander off to do something else after your fifteen minutes off, set a timer to remind you to get back on course.

Ten-minute rule: Another way to keep on track is to promise yourself that you'll only work on a tedious task for ten minutes. After that, you can quit. More than likely, you will find that once you've started, it's hard to stop, and you'll end up putting in way more time than you thought.

Now you have ideas for managing procrastination. Next, let's look at some specific tips to help you better manage your time.

It's Time to Be on Time

You may think that getting to places on time is hopeless, an impossible goal to achieve, but it can be done. Here are some ideas that many women with ADHD find helpful:

Place alarms in different places: Set several alarms in different places. People with ADHD are notorious for having a hard time waking up in the morning. Try placing an alarm clock next to your bed, another across the room, and a third in your bathroom. Buy the loudest ones you can find—some even shake your bed or fly off the table, forcing you to get up and physically move across the room to turn them off.

Use timers to help with starting/stopping: Set an alarm for the time you need to start a project and set a second alarm to go off when it's time to stop. This is a great way to help you get through the transition from starting to stopping, or cuing you to start on something you've been avoiding, like paperwork, and getting you to stop doing pleasurable activities like browsing the Web or playing computer games.

Avoid doing "one last thing": Get into the habit of not doing that last thing before leaving the house. Sorting through mail or reading the front page of the newspaper will cost you precious time and make you late. And checking your e-mail or Facebook even "just for a quick second" is verboten!

Tricks of the Techie Trade for Timeliness

There are hundreds of gadgets and apps for your smartphone and computer that can help you organize your day, break down tasks, and even hold yourself accountable. Many of them have visual cues, and people with ADHD tend to respond well to visuals. You can go to http://ADDconsults.com to get the names of specific apps available at the Apple store to help you with time management. Computer technology is incredibly helpful in keeping you on track, but there are many things you can do using items you already have in the house.

Outta Sight, Outta My Mind!
Visual Cues as Memory Joggers

The more you utilize systems that are "in your face," the easier it will be to remember what you need to do. Here are some ideas to help you with the daily stuff:

- If you get lost in thought while showering and end up racing to get out the door, try a suction cup clock made specifically for the shower.

- Use a waterproof notepad to capture your most creative moments in the shower.

- Invest in lots and lots of inexpensive clocks and place them throughout your house so you can keep tabs on the time and/or use alarms as needed to stay on track.

- Write down your morning routine, step by step, including how much time is needed per step, on index cards. Tape these cards to your bathroom mirror.

- Use dry erase markers and write your kids' morning and bedtime schedules/routines on their mirrors, or use dry erase boards placed wherever your kids need to have visual reminders.

- Write reminders on the windshield of your car with dry erase markers. Just remember to erase them before you head out!

- Put sticky notes on your dashboard.

- Leave reminder messages for yourself on your cell phone or answering machine, or e-mail reminders to yourself.

- Use temporary tattoos on which you can write short memory joggers. These are available online; just Google "to-do list temporary tattoo."

- Use a big color-coded calendar on your wall right near your family launching pad to record everyone's weekly schedule and appointments. Assign each family member a marker color. This works great for the entire family or for an individual.

There are literally hundreds of ways to help you manage your time. Entire books are written on the topic. But there's more to utilizing such tips. Let's dig a little deeper.

Managing Your Relationship with Time from the Inside Out

We tend to focus on practical solutions to our problems and hope that little tips and tricks will solve all of our woes, but, in reality, resolving the time management issues associated with ADHD issues goes deeper than that—in fact, it goes right to the heart. So you were born with an ADHD brain. It's not a death sentence, but neither is it a dance in the park. Accept that your ADHD will most likely be a lifelong challenge. At times, the symptoms may abate, and you'll go merrily through life. But life circumstances, and even your own biology, can make symptoms worse. Be prepared for the ups and downs in life, just like everyone else. Sometimes you'll hit on a tactic that works for you, but often it won't work forever. Don't give up! There is no need to chastise yourself when things go wrong. You aren't weak or incapable. Use your creativity and innate resources to search for new ways to manage things that get in the way of succeeding or feeling good about yourself. Somewhere, somehow, you will know what they are and how to find your way.

If you're brave enough to stop, slow down, and take just three minutes to read this, it could change everything. Look inward to find out what is at the root of your procrastination and how it makes you feel. You've been so rushed, so stressed, that you've spent your whole life looking outward at piles, your watch, your empty pantry, and unfinished projects, allowing yourself to be overcome by your perceived failures, listening to those old tapes in your head of how you "shoulda, coulda, woulda." Stop right now and let yourself feel. Listen to your gut. What is it telling you?

Deeper Solutions to Procrastination

Take a deep breath, listen to how you're feeling, and then move forward with these new tools in your toolbox. Even little tricks can make a big difference.

Spell It Out

When you find yourself in spinout mode, use acronyms to help you get out of your chaotic inner state. You can even jot them down on index cards and post them where you'll likely need to see them, such as your kitchen, work, or home office. Here are some examples:

- STOP
  - Stop.
  - Take a long, deep breath.
  - Observe your gut feelings.
  - Proceed onward.
- SOS: Stop Obsessing, Silly!

You can use these acronyms or make some up that work for you. They can help you to stop your mental spinout and become calm and refocused.

Mega Mantras

Mega mantras (my term) are phrases repeated to yourself to help you move through an area of difficulty. When I'm avoiding exercise or chores that I detest, I use this one, and it's literally changed my life: *Don't do it because you have to, do it because you can.* In other words, I reframe the situation. Instead of being annoyed, I feel grateful that I have the ability to get out and jog or that I have a washing machine to make laundry chores easier. Come up with your own phrases to help you jump into activities you've been avoiding and feel thankful for your good fortune. Shifting the way you think about a task can help you move forward.

It can be hard to stop, think, and then proceed in the direction that is best for you, but, with practice, it can be done. Learning how to use your time in optimal ways by using planners and other time management systems is all part of developing time management skills. Give yourself time to get into new patterns and habits. They won't start working overnight, but once you get the hang of them, you will be amazed and pleased at how much more you get done—and, just as important, how much better you'll feel. Now that you have some practical tips and helpful insights for managing your time and taming procrastination, let's take a look at yet another area of challenge for many women with ADHD—clothing!

CHAPTER 5

Clothing Loathing

The day had arrived for Liz to attend her favorite aunt's sixtieth birthday party. She had twenty minutes left to get dressed. *Where is that invitation, anyway?* she thought. *Did it say what the dress code is? I don't know if I have anything appropriate, let alone clean. Everyone else knows how to put a stupid outfit together. Why can't I?* Liz grabbed skirts and blouses in a panic, trying on various outfits as sweat gathered on her forehead. *Why did I wait until the last minute again? I hate this! I'm going to make a fool out of myself. I just know it.* Nothing looked right. Finally, she chose a simple black dress. Then she noticed the yogurt stain near the collar. She crumpled to the floor in a heap, banged her fist on her closet door, and burst into tears. Figuring it wasn't worth all the trouble to go to a "dumb" birthday party, she quickly called her aunt and told her a bald-faced lie about having suddenly come down with something. Then guilt climbed on her lap and cuddled up with shame, and the three of them had their own little pity party. Again.

Clothing: The "X Files" for Women with ADHD

Something as seemingly simple as putting together an outfit can be an agonizing task if you have ADHD. Again, it requires the executive function of being able to select and prioritize a few items out of many and to be able to see which items go together. You might also become overwhelmed while shopping for clothes, just like at the grocery store, with hundreds of items distracting you. Procrastination may also play a role in tripping you up when you're trying to get ready for an event. And since many women with ADHD have weight problems due to eating disorders, chances are you have an array of different-sized clothes in your closet, making it hard to find the right size to wear. These are just a few of the myriad of challenges women with ADHD face.

Mirror, Mirror on the Wall…?

You might also struggle with self-esteem issues relating to your appearance. Perhaps as a young girl you commonly heard criticisms from other girls because you, like many children with ADHD, were "out of step" socially, including with the latest clothing fads. Maybe you've carried this insecurity about how you look—or should look—into adulthood, making clothing choices an area of anxiety and avoidance. You may be intensely self-conscious due to a lifetime of perceived "failures" in other areas, so this just adds to the pile. Since how you dress is a veritable sandwich board of your identity, putting yourself on display "for the world" to judge can be daunting indeed, especially if your sense of self is already vulnerable.

Closet of Chaos

I'd be willing to bet $100 that the closets of nine out of ten women with ADHD are nothing short of a disaster zone. Impulsivity comes into play here, as do shopping addictions and forgetfulness. How many white blouses do you really need? Did you forget you already have an orange purse that's been sitting in its shopping bag on the floor of your closet for the last six months? Overshopping coupled with organizational challenges almost always leads to clutter. Visual overload ·then makes it harder to find appropriate outfits when blouses, slacks, and more have multiplied in your closet. Finally, procrastination makes it hard to *start* organizing your closet, and hyperfocus makes it hard to *stop*, causing the whole process to be stressful.

Fabric Phobic

Remember the story "The Princess and the Pea"? The princess lay awake all night unable to sleep because she was irritated by the pea she felt under twenty mattresses and twenty featherbeds. Many women with ADHD can identify with the poor princess, for they, too, seem to be intensely sensitive to everything tactile. Women's clothing, often fitted and tight, feels constricting and suffocating. Seams in socks and underwear can be excruciating. Certain fabrics like wool or polyester are verboten, not only for their discomfort, but because they can cause rashes on sensitive skin. In a *Psychiatry Investigation* article, Ghanizadeh (2011) states that "ADHD and sensory problems may occur together and interact," and that "sensory processing problems in children with ADHD are more common than in typically developing children." *Sensory overresponsivity* is a heightened negative response to sensory (such as visual, auditory, or tactile) input. People who have this are overly sensitive and reactive to stimuli. Another article on the subject, written by Bröring and colleagues (2008), shows that more girls than boys with ADHD suffer from *tactile defensiveness*, a negative response to certain types of touch and textures. It makes sense that these tactile sensitivities continue as you grow into adulthood, with sensitivity to fabric being just one of many. Since having hypersensitivities is one of a dozen problems for you related to clothing, it follows that shopping, where you need to try on outfit after outfit, can be a painful experience, one that you'd prefer to avoid.

Just as with cooking, not all women with ADHD struggle with these issues. Some are brilliant at fashion and dressing themselves beautifully.

But over the years, many women have talked to me about their challenges in this area.

So, I Either Wear All Black or Go Naked, Right?

Short of going Goth or getting arrested for indecent exposure, there are lots of practical, doable suggestions to help women with ADHD organize their closets, coordinate outfits, manage clothing clutter, do laundry, and even shop for clothes. These activities, though not always pleasant, can certainly be made less unpleasant. Consider the following tips on organizing and managing your clothes.

Organizing Your Closet

Facing your closet can feel like looking at a psychedelic spinning explosion of colors, textures, and fabrics, especially if you're short on space. How do you organize your clothes when you're looking at a sea of fabric? It can all be overwhelming, but once you come up with some strategies, you may find that the closet isn't a scary place after all.

The magical storage bin: A closet can easily become cluttered if you haven't come up with a system for organizing your belongings. One simple solution for managing an overstuffed closet is to store out-of-season clothes in another closet in your house. If that's not an option, put them in long, stackable plastic storage bins, which can be placed on shelves above your current seasonal clothes in your closet, under your bed, or even in a dry, safe spot in your basement.

The old hanger trick: Do you have a hard time deciding which clothes to keep and which to give away? Making such choices based on frequency of use can be most helpful. To do this, you can use the old hanger trick. Arrange all the clothes in your closet with the hanger tip facing away from you. After you've worn an item, hang it back up with the hanger tip facing toward you. After one year, note which hanger tips are still facing away from you. Those are items you haven't worn in a year. If you haven't worn them in a year, there is likely a reason. Perhaps they don't fit, are out of style, or are just not you anymore and need to be removed from your closet. Give them to charity or to friends, because they're taking up precious space.

Bonus Tips

There are hundreds of other ways to manage clutter in the closet. Below are more tips to help you tame your closet and your clothes:

- Store out-of-season clothes in otherwise empty suitcases.

- Use hanging clear plastic or vinyl shoe storage bags for purses, scarves, and jewelry and hang them on the inside of your closet door so that you can easily see what's in them.

- Utilize dead space: Shoe organizers can go under hanging garments. Add shelves higher up on the walls for T-shirts, jeans, and sweaters.

- Mount a pegboard in your closet for necklaces, scarves, and purses.

- Store purses on hooks slipped over the closet rod.

- Consider labeling shelves of stacked folded pieces (such as long-sleeved T-shirts) to make it easier to find and store them.

- Assemble whole outfits on hangers, with accessories hanging over the top. Narrow these outfits down by function (business, social) and style (casual, supercasual, fancy).

- Organize stacked items like T-shirts and sweaters so it's easier to find them—say, by color.

- Set up zones: blouses in one section, slacks in another, or work clothes in one section and casual wear in another.

- Organize hanging items by color.

There are plenty of ways to organize your closet. What's important is to use systems that work for *you*.

Outrunning the "Perfect Outfit" Gauntlet

As simple and even pleasurable as it may be for many women, for a woman with ADHD, coordinating an outfit can feel like assembling a five-hundred-piece jigsaw puzzle with a blindfold on and a gun to her head. Here are a few tips, however, that can help reduce the stress and improve the outcome.

Find stores that organize by color and style: When shopping, find clothing stores that organize their items by color and style so that you can easily choose pieces that go together. These stores have websites or catalogs, so you may have the added benefit of seeing outfits on models, giving you an idea of what look to go for. For the woman with ADHD who hates all laundry-related chores, including ironing, you can also find clothes that are wrinkle free. For a list of my favorite online retailers and catalogs, visit my website at http://ADDconsults.com.

Create records of outfits that work: Tired of having to reinvent the wheel every time you're invited to a social or business event? Use index cards to note what outfit you've worn for each event you attend. For example, for a formal evening wedding in August, note the outfit and accessories and write the occasion, date, weather, and other pertinent details on the top of the card. Keep your cards in your closet in a decorative box or in a simple folder labeled "outfits." In lieu of the index cards, you can take photos of your completed outfits laid out (or shoot a photo of yourself in the mirror) and organize the photos by category on your phone or upload them to your computer. You can name the folders things like "work," "summer evening events," "conferences," "skiing vacations," and so on. The index cards or photos will give you a quick verbal or visual record so that you don't have to start from scratch every time you need to dress for a particular type of occasion.

Use a minimalist palette: It's also easier to put outfits together if you use a minimalist palette. Choose two neutral colors per season for the bulk of your outfits, and then select a few accent colors.

Select outfits before you need them: Always select outfits for yourself, and for your kids if you have them, the night before to avoid last-minute scurrying and to be sure you have something clean, ironed, and presentable. If the clothes aren't prone to wrinkling, you can even put the entire outfit on one hanger and place it on your (or your kids') doorknob the night before. That will make it easy to fetch the next morning before you dash off to work or school. Another option, if your children's clothes are not prone to wrinkling, is to put your kids to bed wearing the clothes they'll wear the next day. This is a great way to avoid the morning rush.

Create reminders to dry-clean outfits: After wearing an outfit that you know will need a trip to the dry cleaner, put it aside (or better, in your car). This will help remind you to get it cleaned so that it will be ready to wear next time you reach for it.

Consider purchasing lots of socks and "uniforms": To avoid agonizing over assembling outfits and to cut down on laundry time, purchase a lot of the same items, such as jeans, socks, and underwear. If you're comfortable with the concept of having your own daily uniform of sorts, this will work! After all, Einstein rarely wore suits but reportedly had a number of identical gray suits so he wouldn't have to decide, and he favored wearing a loose-fitting cotton sweater, going sockless, and wearing sandals. Steve Jobs wore his own "uniform"—a black mock turtleneck, jeans, and sneakers—and Mark Zuckerberg, cofounder of Facebook, stated in a *Forbes* article that he owns "maybe about twenty identical gray T-shirts" (Smith 2012). Actress Jamie Lee Curtis told the American Association of Retired Persons (AARP), "I wear only black and white...I own one pair of blue jeans" (quoted in Alvarez 2008). If these high-profile people can simplify their wardrobes, perhaps you can, too!

We've just looked at helpful ways for you to organize and manage clothes that you already have. But when you need new clothes, how can you find outfits that really work for *you*? How can you find outfits that feel good and fit well—that is, clothes that "succeed" for you? When you have ADHD, "dressing for success" takes on a whole new meaning, so let's see how you can do it!

Dressing for Success

If you have tactile sensitivity, you have numerous options. These may not put you on *Vogue*'s runway, but they will at least keep you feeling comfortable in your own skin. You will need to experiment with various options. Are you more comfortable wearing tightly fitted clothes or something loose fitting and roomy? Some women prefer heavy blankets on their beds as the weight offers a calming effect, while others find that less is more and feel suffocated under the bulk of bed covers. The same holds true with clothing. This can get tricky when dressing for the workplace and special outings where you can't get away with wearing comfy, lived-in sweats! Some stores specialize in soft clothing and carry items for both business and casual wear. They even rate their products on a scale from 1 to 3 according to softness. Go to http://ADDconsults.com for a list of these stores.

Other stores offer a wide range of fuller-cut clothes, many made with softer, silkier fabrics, and have selections grouped by color and style so that it's much easier for the indecisive, overwhelmed ADHD shopper to choose outfits that go together. You can find a list of stores that offer such clothing items at http://ADDconsults.com.

Nearly every woman with ADHD I've talked to has expressed an intense hatred for wool and certain synthetic fabrics, such as spandex, polyester, and rayon. They don't like stiff clothes or panty hose either. Tactile sensitivity rules, so finding comfortable fabrics, styles, and cuts will help you live in your own (covered) skin. As the late, great comedienne Gilda Radner once said, "I base most of my fashion taste on what doesn't itch."

Shoes, too, can be problematic. Since many women with ADHD have the added challenge of being distracted and inattentive, it's helpful to find shoes that not only are comfortable but also don't pose the threat of tripping! I find that flat shoes are always a safer way to go, and these days there are many cute styles to choose from. My own solution for dealing with tactile sensitivities is to wear clothes a size larger than I am. When I'm in super stay-at-home casual mode, I wear men's T-shirts, which are typically more full in cut and tend to be softer. And if I must wear something that is irritating, like sweaters or scratchy linen blouses, I'll wear a soft T-shirt underneath to give my skin a barrier. Here are some other tips:

- When relaxing at home, find sweatpants with a nonbinding or drawstring waistband, oversized sweatshirts, and gym shoes with a wide toe (or sandals).

- Look for *soft, soft, soft* clothing. Fleece is a winter favorite. One hundred percent cotton and jersey are also easy on the skin.

- "No seam" socks are available online. (See http://ADDconsults .com for specific websites.)

- You can also wear underwear and socks inside out to avoid seams touching your skin.

- If necklaces make you feel like you're choking, wear a light scarf instead, or wear a pin to dress up your outfit.

- Remove labels and tags from your clothes! Cutting or ripping them out can leave a jagged edge that creates even more physical discomfort. Try using a seam ripper to remove the tag or use no-sew hemming tape to tack it down.

- Some women report that they feel calmer and more comfortable wearing snug-fitting items against their skin (the sensation is similar to using heavy blankets). Consider wearing a bathing suit or body suit that snaps at the crotch under your clothes, or wear layers of clothes to provide the weight your body might crave.

- Check your laundry detergent! Use nonscented gentle brands and add nonscented softener. Prewashing new clothes multiple times often helps with scratchiness.

- Elastic waistbands can be a lifesaver, but only if the added stretch makes you feel less constricted compared to a regular waistband.

- Many women with ADHD dislike boat or scoop necks and V-necks. Crew necks are often preferred but may not be stylish enough in certain situations, so consider layering with different necklines.

But finding clothes that don't make you squirm in discomfort is just part of the shopping challenge. You still have to physically get yourself through the store and navigate the highly stimulating mall environment.

Getting in the Shopping Groove

There's no getting around it—you simply have to buy new clothes. Here are some tips to make it a bit more pleasant for you:

- Plan ahead. Shop on days when you are feeling good. Don't go when you're irritable, tired, or rushed. Set it up in your planner as you would any other appointment.

- Find quieter clothing stores that are easy on your senses, where the clothes aren't all jammed together and there's lots of "breathing room." Often these are boutiques rather than big-name stores at malls.

- Look for stores with "kinder" lighting versus fluorescent bulbs.

- Shop at stores that have a lot of cotton clothes.

- Consider buying used clothes, which are often softer, having been washed and worn.

- Find smaller shops where you can get individual attention and/ or personal shoppers. Note the name of your salesperson so you can use that person the next time you visit.

- Bring a friend, sister, or daughter and let her "play Barbie." Many women love pulling outfits together and would enjoy helping you. In exchange, treat her to lunch.

- Consider shopping online or via catalogs to avoid sensory overload.

- Take clothes home to try on. This is helpful if you need extra time and hate feeling rushed, or you don't like the store's lighting, dressing rooms, or general commotion. Return the items you don't like or that don't fit.

Now you've got some tools for choosing outfits under your belt. But once you've got the clothes, you have to keep them clean, so let's see how to make laundry a less painful chore.

Beating the Laundry Blues

Remember that doing laundry also involves healthy executive functioning. The same challenges of sorting, following a sequence of steps, keeping track of time, and dealing with distractions, boredom, and forgetfulness are all in play. Not having clean underwear or not being able to find two matching socks can add a lot of stress to your daily routine. Add a child, or two, or more, and you have double or triple the amount of work and stress when it comes to managing laundry. On top of keeping up with the laundry, which is difficult for many, you may—because of sensory sensitivities—have to comb the market aisles for unscented, hypoallergenic products, compounding the problem.

There are many ways to manage your laundry, but the best way is to find the system that works best for *you*...not what worked best for your mom or grandmother. Below are some general ideas to help address all the typical ADHD issues that come with each and every load.

Have two laundry baskets or bins: one for whites and one for colors. If you have a partner and/or children, have a pair of baskets for each person. Put the bins or baskets wherever you are most likely to disrobe. Get an attractive one if it's going in a room other than the bedroom, bathroom, or laundry room. And be realistic. If you take off your clothes while watching TV, then put your baskets in the TV room! The containers don't have to be fancy hundred-dollar ones. You can get baskets or bins for around ten bucks. Another tip to cut down on sorting is to buy all your socks in the same color and style. For a family, do this for each person to keep the sock-eating monster at bay. If your children are fairly close in age, buy the same size and color socks and underwear and just divvy them up. This simplifies the whole laundry process.

Hate to iron? Do you put it off until the last minute and then find that you're covered in wrinkles? No worries. Take your hair dryer and blow the wrinkles right off of you. (Be careful, though, if you're wearing the clothes—it's easy to burn yourself.) This works best on lighter weight fabrics. Also, some dryers have a steam cycle that dewrinkles clothes. If yours has one, enjoy your new "iron"! (Just be sure to pull the clothes out right when the cycle ends—or you'll be back to wrinkled square one.)

When Laundry Is Out of Sight, It's Definitely Out of Mind!

Does your nose remind you that you've left the laundry sitting in the washer for three days? To avoid the "stinky, clean clothes syndrome," consider the tips below.

Using a timer is a fantastic way to help you manage every stage of washing and drying your clothes. You can set the timer on your oven or program your smartphone or computer to remind you when it's time to move clothes from the washer to the dryer. There are even washers and dryers with a "snooze alarm" that keeps going off until you open the door and move your laundry from the washer to the dryer or take it out of the dryer. You can also use a *mega mantra* (word, sound, or phrase repeated to aid concentration in meditation), such as "Laundry, laundry, gotta do the laundry," to help you remember the various stages.

Making Peace with Routine

"Aaaack!" you yell, "Not *routine*! That's boring!" For the woman with ADHD, the word "routine" may sound like a four-letter word. True, repetition and routine may not offer the creative juice and stimulation you crave, but with routine comes peace of mind both from having done the dreaded chores and from following a system that keeps you on track and moving forward. By sticking with a routine, you'll spend far less time scrambling for clean clothes or dashing to the laundry room, rushing to get things washed at the last minute. Who knows? The lack of anxiety and stress might make you even more productive! Again, figure out what works best for you. You might do laundry once a week—say, every Sunday—or perhaps you find it best to do a load or two each day so you don't get overwhelmed. Or, you can "twin" this chore with another activity—for example, throwing in laundry before watching your favorite TV show. Twinning will help remind you that it's laundry time.

Doing the Dirty Laundry Hop

Just like dancing, laundry has steps you must follow. Following steps can be tough for a woman with ADHD, so here are a few tips. Write each step of your laundry routine onto large index cards or on a poster board, and then hang the cards or board on the laundry room wall. It might look like this:

1. Make three piles:
    - Whites (hot water and maybe bleach, if needed)
    - Mediums/bold colors (warm water)
    - Darks (cold water)

    (Hint: I wash most clothes in cold except for underwear, socks, and towels/linens.)

2. Wash underwear and socks first. (Remember the triage approach? Most important first!)

3. Throw in dryer when done.

4. Wash jeans, work clothes, shirts.

5. Hang to dry or throw in dryer.

6. Wash towels and sheets.

7. Throw in dryer when done.

8. Sort, fold, and put away socks, underwear, and other items of clothing. (You may need a trigger to remind you to put clothes away, if they tend to sit in baskets for days. Maybe make it a point to put away your clothes before moving into a pleasant activity, like going online, talking on the phone, or watching TV.)

9. Fold towels and sheets and place in linen closet.

You will have your own system, and perhaps yours will differ from the one above. That's fine. Just try to be consistent so that it becomes second nature. That way you don't have to reinvent washing day. These are just a few tips to help you master your laundry chores. The important thing is to find what works for you and stick to your routine. But what if you absolutely *hate* routine?

Roll Away Your Resistance Blocks

Laundry is tedious. It's a never-ending monster chore that never goes away. And since it is repetitive and boring (for most), you probably resist facing it. After all, most women with ADHD find boring routines nearly impossible to manage because there are so many other, fun things to do! The next time you're ready to put clean clothes away but find yourself frozen at the thought of how *looooong* it will take and how *boooor-ing* it is, time yourself. More than likely, the time involved is much less than it seems (partly because boring tasks *seem* to take longer than they do). Once you realize that putting clothes away takes, say, fifteen minutes instead of an hour, think of when you can fit a fifteen-minute task into your day (or week). Write it in your planner, or program it into your computer or smartphone. Or follow the old Mary Poppins adage that a spoonful of sugar helps the medicine go down. Crank up the stereo with your favorite music while putting laundry away, or fold your laundry while watching one of your favorite TV shows.

To entice children to put dirty laundry in bins, be creative! Purchase a laundry bag that doubles as a basketball net and place it over the bedroom door. Your children will love playfully tossing their clothes into the net, which keeps clothes off the floor. And by all means, if you have children capable of doing their own laundry, let them!

One of the biggest complaints I hear from women is that they are frustrated by family members, including themselves, who habitually pick out clean, folded clothes from the laundry basket. As a result, the newly folded clothes never even land in drawers! Wouldn't it be nice if your family members could take care of their own clothes instead of you having to pick up after them, especially when it's so difficult to manage your own clothes? If you feel frazzled at the sight of heaps of clean clothes in baskets but can't seem to put them away, get to the bottom of why that is. Is it not knowing where to put things? Are there too many things to put away? Is it boredom? Lack of time? Break down your reasons one by one, and then you can figure out strategies to help manage the problem. Again, many clutter and/or organizing problems can be solved by first going inward and identifying the stress triggers.

Whether it's clothes shopping, choosing outfits to wear, organizing and washing your clothes, or struggling with tactile discomfort, remind yourself that though these activities might seem easy for other women to manage—and even enjoy—you certainly aren't alone in finding the whole thing challenging and unpleasant. Your ADHD neurobiology is again reminding you to find ways to make these demands of daily living less painful and stressful.

CHAPTER 6

When Mommy Has ADHD

Eight-year-old Jake charged through the front door, slamming it behind him. Finding his mother, Liz, reading the paper in the den, he planted his feet in front of her, shaking in rage, his face bright red. "The coach said I can't play on the soccer team because *you* never sent in the paperwork. You promised you'd make a doctor's appointment for me to get the physical filled out but…" Jake was so furious, he started to cry in frustration.

Liz trembled as she tried to console Jake, but she couldn't find the words. Not only had she forgotten to call the doctor, she'd also misplaced the forms. Her face burned in shame; her heart was broken for having disappointed her son, letting him down once again with her forgetfulness. Liz felt herself being pulled into yet another depression, her guilt and shame overwhelming her.

Do as I Say, Not as I Do

If you are a mother with ADHD, perhaps you've asked yourself these questions: *Why doesn't my poor kid have a better mom? How can I manage my child's disorganization when I can't even handle my own? How do I help my child with homework when I procrastinate with my own daily chores?* And worse, maybe you feel it's hard to even connect with your child at times when you're off in "la-la land." Sari Solden, MS (2007, 1), ADHD expert and best-selling author of *Women with Attention Deficit Disorder*, describes the dilemma succinctly:

> Consider the job description of homemaker and child-care giver: You're required to provide all the organization and structure for three or more people. Tasks are poorly defined, filled with distractions, and require constant multitasking. Because much of the work, including cooking, cleaning, and laundry, is boring, you must be able to function without needing a high level of interest or stimulation.
>
> Appearance is important as well: You must create an attractive household, attending to the details of décor and the children's clothing. It is also important to maintain a calm demeanor while caring for children, who, by definition, have problems with attention and behavior.

Many women with ADHD say that it's harder to stay at home with kids than to be a "working" mom. And raising children when you have ADHD is beyond challenging, but it kicks the stress up a notch when one or more of your children also have ADHD.

The Gene Doesn't Fall Far from the Parent

ADHD is often passed down genetically, so it is not at all uncommon for a woman with ADHD to have one or more kids with ADHD. A 1996 study by Biederman and colleagues states that "strongly increased risks for ADHD (57%) among the offspring of adults with ADHD have been reported" (343). Such a scenario leads to the proverbial "blind leading the blind" when a mother with ADHD tries to teach her child the very things she struggles with herself on a daily basis. Though ADHD symptoms are primarily the same in both children and adults, they differ in how they manifest. Let's see how the most common ADHD symptoms compare in you and your child with ADHD and the outcomes they present.

The "Last Minute" Adrenaline Hit

Procrastination is one of the more common ADHD symptoms, but it's also one of the most challenging. Your child may wait until the last minute to hand in homework, whereas you may put off completing an assignment for work. For both of you, the adrenaline "anxiety rush" is often the stimulant that forces you to get your projects done, but, unfortunately, the finished product may suffer.

But Mommy, School Is So Bo-o-o-o-oring!

Inattention is another common ADHD symptom seen in both child and adult. If your child isn't paying attention in school, she might miss important information for a school project, resulting in a poor grade. As an adult, you might forget to sign your child's school papers, pack his lunch, or make regular dental appointments. You may not even notice that he's outgrown his clothes and his ankles are showing below his pants or that your daughter hasn't had her allowance in three weeks.

Mommy, Are You Listening?

Your child might also be affected by your inattention. Sadly, this inattention can cause you and your child to have a "disconnect." For example, if you're spending hours in "high-stim" computer land, your child might interpret that as you not caring about him. This can create significant issues within your relationship, such as perceived feelings of rejection—for example, "Mom doesn't really care about me. She's more interested in her computer game." Your child may experience depression from feeling rejected and/or act out to get your attention. This may result in low self-esteem due to your not being "up" on his activities, such as not remembering to attend his sporting events or forgetting to have his special outfits for these events clean and ready.

Jumping off the Deep End... Without a Paddle

Impulsivity is acting without thinking about consequences. A boy may impulsively push the kid in front of him in a school line whereas a woman might overdraw her checking account because of impulsive purchases. As a mom, you might have a terrible time setting up schedules for your kids and following them. Or maybe you've blurted out something you wish you hadn't, hurting your child's feelings.

When Mom Is the Energizer Bunny

Like impulsivity, hyperactivity can also get in the way of positive parenting. If you are hyperactive, how do you connect if your child prefers quiet board games and watching TV? Children with ADHD may find it impossible to sit still in class, whereas a hyperactive mom might have no patience for a quiet, introspective child who wants her mom to read with her in bed at night, or go to plays, movies, or other activities that require slowing down and paying attention. The child might interpret this as the mom not caring.

Too Much, Too Loud, Too Annoying

Children make messes and are typically loud and demanding. This puts tremendous stress on you if you are overreactive and/or hypersensitive. If your fuse is short, you may lash out at family members for every little misstep, whereas overreactive children might cry at even the most minor setback, like not being able to tie their shoes. And as much as you love your child, you might hate having her climb, tug, and poke at you if you are hypersensitive. Shrieking laughter and crying might put you over the top, making you feel inadequate because you feel that you are intolerant of normal child behaviors.

The Quicksand of Low Self-esteem

The challenges of parenting with ADHD can drag your self-esteem down into the swamp of depression. Thoughts like *Why can't I be a better mom?* or *What's wrong with me that I can't even get dinner on the table?* may trigger guilt, anger, and shame. You may be glared at for being a "bad mother" because you can't control your kids' behavior in public. Others may criticize you for not being able to keep up the house. Your children may feel ashamed to have friends over and, as a result, become socially isolated. They may develop anxiety or compensate for your so-called deficits or forgetfulness by taking on additional responsibilities, like tidying up or reminding you of upcoming events, which makes you feel even worse.

In general, moms with ADHD typically feel overwhelmed and question their ability to parent effectively. But there are ways you can make life easier for you and your children. Now that you have a better understanding of how your ADHD might make parenting difficult, especially if your child has ADHD as well, let's look at some of them.

Making Life Easier: There Is Hope!

Despite all the challenges, being a mom with ADHD is not all gloom and doom. Impulsive moms can also create a home full of fun adventures and spontaneous activities and outings. They may encourage creativity and trying new things. In their 2011 book, *Driven to Distraction*, ADHD experts Dr. Edward Hallowell and Dr. John Ratey state, "Creativity is impulsivity gone right" (219). Let's dive in and look at some tips to help you reduce the stress of parenting.

Turning "Ordealtime" into Mealtime

Now is the time to tune out your mother's or grandmother's voice in your head about what dinner is "supposed" to be like. Mealtime is successful only when it works for your particular family. If you have a child with ADHD, the rules must change. Though ideally you'd like your children to sit quietly every night with the whole family, sometimes that's just not possible. If your child is significantly hyperactive and simply cannot sit still long enough to enjoy a family dinner, consider allowing your fidgety child to stand up while eating or sit on a bouncy ball. And if it's *you* who has a hard time sitting still long enough to enjoy a meal with your family and pay attention to everyone's chatter about their day, you might benefit by using small hand fidgets like a squishy ball to keep yourself calm or taking a brisk walk before dinner to discharge some of your energy. You might also want to discuss adjusting your meds with your doctor so that the meds are still working for you during this important part of your and your family's day.

Timing Is Everything

Many children with ADHD who are on stimulant medication often have little appetite until later in the evening when their meds wear off. Many experience *rebound,* which means a worsening of symptoms and/or irritability, as their medications wear off. If forcing your child to sit at the dinner table causes stress or worse, consider allowing him to eat dinner later in a quiet room, even perhaps in front of the TV. Family dinners can be too stimulating, and expecting him to sit quietly may simply be too much for him. And for those who come home from school starving for the same reason (meds have worn off), why not give your child an early dinner? Then she can join the family at their meal for a short period of time and leave if needed. She can even join up for dessert if she's eaten her meal earlier.

Of course, not all children have ADHD. If your children do not, it may be *you* who gets overwhelmed at the dinner table because, after all, kids are still kids, ADHD or not. Another tip is to feed the children before you have dinner. You can simply sit and chat with your family about their day and then serve yourself (and your partner) later on when it's quieter. Setting a relaxing tone with soft music can also help temper the excitability of loud children. To bend the rules even more, it might help to calm things down by having a TV on. This will give the children something other than a wild ruckus to focus their attention on. The result? Calmer meals for all of you.

When You Want to Hide Under the Table

Believe it or not, there *are* ways to enjoy a peaceful dinner. Perhaps the ideas here will work well for you and your family. Planning ahead of time so that you're not rushing through meal preparation will help immensely. If your situation is not like the one above, and having the TV on is not helpful but rather creates *more* stimuli and havoc, turn off the TV and phones to help make things calmer. "Jiffy" meals that require little prep time are not a luxury but a real solution to a real problem. Enlist the help of your partner and/or your kids to manage this hectic time of day. If your child has ADHD or other challenges, make the chore fit his capabilities and mood. Maybe he can be in charge of clearing the table or wiping down the counter.

Going to the Head of the Class

Just like mealtime, school demands can also make a mom with ADHD want to jump off a cliff at times. It's hard enough for you to keep track of your own responsibilities: work, keeping the home in shape, planning holidays, setting up appointments, shopping, and so much more. How do you also balance your child's needs in school? Here are some tips to help you stay on top of things.

Taking the Fight out of Homework Time

I'm guessing that you and your child go head to head when it comes to homework. I hear this all the time from moms with ADHD and experienced it firsthand with my own child. Parents feel obligated to make sure their child is being responsible, but for a mom with ADHD, that can seem harder than the homework itself. Your relationship with your child is far more important than homework, so if homework is getting in the way, and you find yourself fighting and stressing over it, find a high school or college student to come in and replace you as the homework dictator. A good tutor can help your child develop strategies in this area and can offer you tips on how to best support your child.

Advocating for Your ADHD Child at School

If your child has ADHD (or other special needs), he may be eligible to receive special services at school. Not all children with ADHD qualify, so it's important to talk to your child's teacher or go directly to the special education director in your district. Many parents are uneasy about disclosing their child's ADHD to school officials. They worry that colleges will reject their child if they see she has been getting special services due to her ADHD. However, in most cases, *not* disclosing the child's ADHD means not getting services that may allow your child to succeed. And often the outcome of nondisclosure is poorer grades and a frustrated child whose self-esteem takes a beating. The more successful your child is now, the more successful she'll be in college. By law, a college cannot discriminate against a student who has a disability, and, again, ADHD is a disability under the Americans with Disabilities Act (ADA).

Getting help for your child in school is a daunting process for all parents, but especially for moms with ADHD. You may get overwhelmed with the amount of paperwork, the frequency of meetings, and the need to track progress. It's always a good idea to stay in close contact with teachers. One simple way is to trade e-mail addresses so that communication is fast and easy. If you do have to attend Individualized Education Plan (IEP) or 504 meetings (these ensure special services or accommodations for your child), it's best to hire a parent advocate who can support you through the entire process. Go to http://ADDconsults.com for info on how to find a parent advocate at the Council of Parent Attorneys and Advocates (COPAA) or the National Disability Rights Network.

Sometimes it's even necessary to hire a disabilities attorney if you aren't able to negotiate with the school to get appropriate supports and services for your child. Attorneys are listed by state at the COPAA website at http://www.copaa.org.

Data In/Data Out

If your child's papers are not getting back to school with your signature because you have lost them or forgotten about them, consider using two folders for your child's survival kit: one for papers coming home that need your attention and one for papers needing to be returned to school. Label them "For Home" and "For School," or whatever works best for you. Take action immediately—read, sign, write a check, or whatever you need to do—and then place the paper in the "For School" folder. And if you have more than one child, have a set of folders for each child. Label each folder with the child's name. To simplify the system even more, consider color-coding the folders—for example, red for "stop, take action"; green for "go back to school."

This is an all-around good system to make sure assignments, projects, and teacher/parent communications are taken care of. But what if, despite your best efforts, your child continues to get into trouble due to missing homework or papers? Should you reveal your ADHD to the teachers?

To Speak or Not to Speak

In my experience, unfortunately, many teachers either don't understand ADHD or don't even believe it exists. Or they may have the attitude that you should be able to "get over it" and handle things by buckling down and acting like the mature adult that you are. Rather than use the term "ADHD," it's much better to describe your difficulties—for example: "I'm a busy person and often find myself disorganized and unable to find my child's papers that need to be signed. Can we work out a better way to communicate about his homework assignments [or school activities or whatever] so that I'm sure to get them back to you in time?"

Or "My memory isn't what it used to be. I don't intentionally forget to get papers back to you, so I apologize. If you don't get them, I'd really, really appreciate it if you could e-mail me a reminder."

The Chore of Getting Kids to Do Chores

As if homework isn't hard enough to stay on top of, how about your child's chores? No one likes to do chores, and moms with ADHD avoid going head to head with their children like the plague. It's simply too exhausting. Consider handing this over to your partner if possible. However, as parents, decide as a team who should do what chores, taking into consideration input from your child. Here are some tips to help lighten the burden.

A Spoonful of Sugar…

Try finding fun ways for your child to do her chores. Rewards work well, though if your child has ADHD, they need to be given immediately. Try writing down chores on small pieces of paper, folding them in half, and tossing them in a bowl or jar. Make it a game to see what task your child will draw. In another bowl, have rewards written down that your child gets to pull out after she completes her chore. Rewards can be an extra hour of TV or computer time, a special outing with a parent, and so on.

Tag Team It

Children often do better when a parent works alongside them. You might turn on fun music and dance with your child as he cleans his room. Don't tell him to clean his room. That's too big. Break it down into doable chunks, such as "Let's first pick up all the clothes and toys from the floor and put them where they belong." Allow yourself to be silly. Make it into a production, with your child the star of the show and you the director. If your child has ADHD, let him listen to music through headphones to stay on task and to prevent distractions. When children are older, let them invite a friend over to help with the big chores in exchange for them heading to the friend's house to help the *friend* out. (Of course, discuss this plan with the child's parent!)

In Plain Sight

Try using a chart to record chores and place check marks next to them as they are completed. Place it in a highly visible spot so both you and your child can stay on top of things. Set aside a specific time every day for your child to do her chores. That will make it easier for both of you to remember.

Pick Your Battles

It may be wise to lower your expectations, as this could make life easier for both you and your child. Is it really necessary that he make his bed every day? If she doesn't clear off the entire table, is it worth fighting over it? Sometimes you may require professional help if things do get out of hand—for example, if your child acts out in ways that can physically or emotionally harm himself or others, especially if he fights with you when you make requests of him. Or perhaps she chronically lies or constantly blames others, and your discipline isn't effective. It's important to find a mental health professional who has a lot of expertise in working with children who have ADHD. There is a professional directory at my website, http://ADDconsults.com; but another great resource for finding someone in your area is Children and Adults with ADHD (CHADD). Call 1-800-233-4050 to connect with the national office. They will give you the number to your local CHADD chapter. The coordinator there will have names of professionals in your area (doctors, therapists, and others) who have expertise in working with children and adults with ADHD. If there isn't a chapter near you, check out the online resource directory at http://www.chadd.org. Above all, don't take it all on yourself by doing everything for your child. Your child needs to learn practical skills at home, and negotiating chores is part of providing positive discipline when raising your child.

Turning "Badtime" into Bedtime

If you are on meds for your ADHD, their effects are probably wearing off just around the time you need them the most: your child's bedtime. You might be experiencing rebound, giving you less patience and reserve. How do you manage?

Consistency Is Calming for Everyone

Children need to know what is expected of them, and bedtime is no different. Be superconsistent with their schedule: TV off at 7:30, bath done by 8:00, lights out at 8:30. That's all easy to say, but as a mom with ADHD, being consistent is typically not in your DNA! If you have a partner, have your partner supervise bath time while you take over bedtime stories. Or take turns, one day on, one day off. If you're a single parent, enlist the help of extended family and friends. Parenting is not for the faint of heart, and when ADHD is in the mix, it's essential to get as much support as possible. Even bringing in a sitter to help you a few times a week with bedtime is well worth the expense. This is often a very vulnerable time for you. The last thing you want to do is engage in an emotional battle with your child. You need your downtime—and she needs her sleep!

Chart It!

Visual cues, again, are extremely helpful because they not only help keep a system going, but take you out of the loop as "the bad guy." Work with your child (if he is old enough) in developing a list of each aspect of the bedtime routine on a small piece of poster board, and tape it to the bedroom or bathroom wall. Kids love check marks. Simply use a printed list with check boxes and instruct your child to mark off each bedtime task once completed. Reward? Extra five minutes of story time, a special morning treat from the treat fairy under his pillow, stickers, or similar fun things.

Winding Down

Many children with ADHD seem to get more wound up at bedtime. If they are on medications, they might be experiencing rebound in which ADHD symptoms worsen. Here are some tips to help everyone relax: Give both yourself and your child downtime before bedtime—no TV, computers, or video games at least an hour before lights out. Offer your child a massage before or after a warm bath, and play calm, soft, relaxing music (such as classical) with no lyrics. Read a book and snuggle.

For some kids, smaller, enclosed spaces or tighter clothing seem to be calming. You can purchase lightweight tents that sit on the bed, giving it a womb-like sensation. Footie pajamas offer the same sensation, as does wearing a one-piece swimsuit or leotard under PJs. There is a product that flashes beams of light onto the ceiling or wall. Your child matches his breathing to the rhythm of the light, allowing him to easily fall asleep. See my website http://ADDconsults.com for specifics on all these products.

When You've Tried Everything

Sometimes nothing works to settle your ADHD child. If this happens frequently, then you may need to call in professional help. Ask your child's pediatrician for ideas, or work with an occupational therapist who can offer a "sensory diet," ways to help your child calm down through a variety of techniques. Your pediatrician should be able to provide you with a referral, or you can consult your closest children's hospital for names.

If Mama Ain't Happy, Ain't Nobody Happy

Many women with ADHD have hypersensitivities and often feel overwhelmed, and parenting challenges can bring these issues to the forefront. If you yell at the kids more often than not or feel a constant sense of despair or even depression, then it's time to take action. Your job as a parent is the toughest one you'll ever have, so it's important that you find ways to de-stress.

Finding Shelter in the Storm

Taking care of yourself has got to be job #1 because no one else can do it for you. If at all possible, spend some time away once a month so you can rejuvenate. Go to a hotel overnight or stay with a friend or family member who doesn't have kids, leaving the children with your partner, a trusted family member, or a sitter. Give yourself a regularly scheduled break. An exhausted mom is not an effective, patient mom. With my own high-energy kids, it took me a long time to accept that I needed to follow this advice in order to save my sanity. I found that going to professional conferences out of state gave me a wonderful break from the stresses of being a parent while also giving me the opportunity to connect with adults who shared my interests and passions.

Mini Time-Outs

Mini time-outs can be lifesavers to help prevent being overwhelmed. When you feel like you're about to explode because your child has triggered you, give yourself a time-out before you do or say something you'll regret. Have your spouse take over while you retreat. Explain this plan ahead of time so your family will understand why you've suddenly disappeared. Not only does this defuse the situation and give you time to calm down, it also serves to model behavior for your child who can then learn how to remove herself during times of stress to calm herself in her room.

Transitioning from your workday to your parenting responsibilities is difficult. After work, stop at a coffee shop to relax and refuel before heading home. Schedule this into your daily routine. If you can't do this, just sitting in your parked car meditating, listening to calming music, or taking a quick nap before going home will make all the difference.

Whether you're a working mom or an at-home mom, enlist the help of babysitters even if you're home. It's imperative to have "me time" so that you can rest, read a book, or head out for a needed break. Just do it!

Many moms neglect their own self-care because they are taking care of others, especially if they have ADHD and they have a child with ADHD. See chapter 11 for more ideas about how to take care of yourself and find the balance you crave. These, again, are all accommodations, not luxuries. You must remove self-blame from your internal dialogue and use these strategies in order to get through some of the hardest years of your life.

Protect Your Self-Esteem Like Gold

Losing your self-esteem because you're struggling every day with your ADHD while trying to meet the demands of caring for your children is not an option. You *can* do something about your sinking sense of self. Becoming proactive and learning self-advocacy skills will help you pull yourself out of a slump and give you a tremendous sense of strength. It doesn't come easy, and it takes time, but you can do it!

Become Your Own Advocate

Educate your spouse, family members, and close friends about your ADHD and how it affects you as a parent. You might consider inviting close family or friends to one of your doctor or therapy appointments so that you can get professional help in supporting your need, your *right*, to be understood.

You might even want to disclose your ADHD to your child's teacher, who can then better understand the school-related difficulties described above. But *only*—and this is a major only—do this if you know for certain that the teacher will be empathetic and encouraging and not criticize you or dismiss your struggles. If the teacher doubts you or denies that ADHD even exists, show the teacher your medical paperwork with your diagnosis (but only if you're comfortable doing so). Ask the teacher to read articles you've printed off the Internet, as much has been written about this topic, or a book on ADHD—perhaps even this book!

Love Yourself by Accepting Help

It can be hard, very hard, to ask for help, but you need to allow yourself to do just that at times and to accept the help offered. What better way to model self-esteem than by telling your child, "It's okay to ask your teacher for help, sweetie," if your daughter encounters difficulties at school?

Working with an ADHD coach or entering therapy with a therapist skilled in working with adults with ADHD will help you put the pieces together as well as understand how your ADHD affects you. Sometimes people need concrete (and professional) help in learning to love themselves.

Say Sayonara to the "Joneses"

Accept that what works for your sister's kids may not work for yours. Stop comparing your situation with hers or with those of others who don't struggle with differences. *Accept* your differences—your ADHD—knowing that this is how your brain is wired and that it's not your fault, nor is it a personality defect or character flaw. To move into healthy self-esteem, you'll need to change expectations of yourself and of your children, bringing those expectations down a notch if needed, in order to be realistic. Part of self-acceptance is learning to forgive yourself during difficult times. "It's my ADHD kicking in" can be another mega mantra to help you hold steady and keep your self-esteem in the healthy zone.

No Woman Is an Island

I can't stress enough that you need both emotional *and* hands-on support. Expect that there will probably be more chaos, disorganization, and tension in your home than in many other people's homes. Avoid "friends" who don't understand your situation or who brag about their "perfect" kids. Keep in mind, too, that outward appearances often don't tell the whole story. These "together" families might be dealing with their own private crises. Find friends who might admit that their kids are challenging, too. Consider befriending other women with ADHD who struggle like you. There are local support groups in many large cities, as well as online support groups. Being a mom with ADHD is often challenging—there's no doubt about that—but it doesn't have to damage your self-esteem. Being aware of your difficulties and finding ways around them can make all the difference. You might find that your ADHD offers you advantages! Your creative thinking, your plethora of interests, and your kind, sensitive soul will outweigh the negatives, as long as you come to a sense of acceptance and move forward with your strengths.

There is no question that living with ADHD is a challenge, and being a mom with ADHD is even more demanding, but using the tips in this chapter can help lighten the burden. You get one shot at parenting your children. You can choose to fall apart, or you can find ways to make this the most exciting part of your life. It certainly is worth the effort.

CHAPTER 7

Stop...in the Name of Love

After a pleasant dinner party with friends one night, Alex popped into her kitchen to refresh the coffee. Her heart skipped a beat when she overheard her boyfriend, Rob, say to his buddy Mark with a chuckle, "Man, I don't know what to do. The truth is that I can't live with her, and I can't live without her. Most of the time, she drives me crazy, but, hell, she puts up with me." She threw down the kitchen towel and ran into the bathroom, choking back tears.

It's one thing for a woman to deal with the consequences of her ADHD, but it adds a whole new dimension when they directly impact her relationships. Many relationship experts have identified their own version of the stages couples go through. Drawing from that research and my own experience, I have identified four main stages of romantic relationships and what they ask of the woman with ADHD. Please note that all couples do not proceed though all four stages, as a couple may split up at any point along the way:

- Stage 1: Getting to Know You

- Stage 2: Getting Serious

- Stage 3: The Honeymoon Is Over

- Stage 4: Mature Love

This list assumes that you meet someone in your twenties and that each stage lasts at least five years. Of course, any time you meet someone new, you start over. We'll begin with the first stage, which ranges from meeting someone new to the early stages of connecting.

Stage 1: Getting to Know You

You may be new to the dating scene—divorced, widowed, old, young, straight, or gay. Regardless of your stage or orientation in life, if you are searching for a romantic partner and you have ADHD, you may experience a whole gamut of challenges above and beyond the typical ones. The issues for the hyperactive subtype are often different than for the inattentive subtype. Impulsivity ranks at the top of the list for the hyperactive subtype, as we'll see below.

Serial Lovers (Kix for Adults)

If you are hyperactive and impulsive, you crave stimuli and abhor boredom. Many hyperactive women stay single and become "serial lovers" because they fear the boredom of being stuck with one partner "till death do us part." Perhaps you've had your share of short sexual flings that have left you feeling empty and raw. The excitement of the roller-coaster ride always ends. Then you pick yourself up off the floor, humiliated and hurt that once again you let your impulsivity take over. If you're the inattentive subtype, however, you have other issues to deal with.

Attraction, Distraction, and Inquisition

If you're the inattentive subtype, when you're first dating, your distractibility may be in high gear. How do you connect with someone with that blaring music from the bar and the whirring fan overhead? What if you keep interrupting, worried you'll forget the point you wanted to get across, not to mention that nagging self-critic in your head who keeps harping on past failures?

The inattentive subtype is often highly self-conscious and overly internal—in short, you're your own personal inquisitor. You might worry incessantly over how you are presenting yourself to your date: *He probably thinks I'm stupid because I can't keep up in conversation or find the right words. Do I look okay? Am I talking enough? Too much?* Your internal dialogue about past relationship failures might also kick in as you worry about "messing things up again" like so many times before.

Stage 2: Getting Serious

Things are heating up, and you're moving into a more serious relationship. You're still on your best behavior, keeping your symptoms just under the surface. But how do you keep up without messing up? You want so much for this to work but are afraid that he will reject you. Unlike a physical disability, your ADHD might be cloaked at first. Then, as you spend more and more time with your new love interest, your symptoms spill out.

Letting the Cat out of the Bag

How do you know when it's time to bring him in on your secret? It can be utterly terrifying to disclose anything that shows your warts and blemishes, but it's important to set the stage for an honest, loving relationship. How do you communicate this to your new love if communication itself brings its own difficulties?

He Said, She Said

Communication is hard enough at times for most couples, but when you add the many symptoms of ADHD to the mix, things can get really tough. In the getting serious phase, the couple begins to share secrets, talk about serious subjects, reveal more of their faults, and take things to a deeper level. Like many women with ADHD, you may struggle with talking about such topics because they can tap into your deeper feelings of insecurity and fear of failure. Because of your anxiety, you may experience chaotic or disorganized thoughts, or you might interrupt, take over the conversation, or shut down completely.

Because your ADHD brain works at the speed of light, you may often be ten steps ahead of your partner in a conversation. You will likely get impatient and want to move forward, often interrupting, partly out of fear that you will forget what you want to say or simply because you are hopelessly bored while waiting for the other person to get to the point. Many women say it feels like being stuck in traffic, and adults with ADHD are notoriously impatient and cannot tolerate traffic jams, waiting in long lines, and similar situations. This can be a real turnoff for your partner.

If all goes well, you and your partner make a commitment to stay together, perhaps through marriage or living together. The excitement and novelty of your new relationship often continues to keep symptoms at bay or at least makes your partner accepting of your unique ways, not realizing that, perhaps down the road, what he finds attractive and interesting may lead to major friction between you. As you will see, patterns begin to change and that's when the problems often begin.

Stage 3: The Honeymoon Is Over

In stage 3, your love is going strong, but the bliss of newly married committed life no longer carries you through the everyday ups and downs. You likely have more responsibilities at work, are adapting to living together, and/or are starting a family—and are doing all this while learning the marital dance of each other's triggers and nuances. As the bills, laundry, and clutter pile up amid sleepless nights with crying babies, important dates are forgotten and tempers get short, adding to the potential for conflict. Such stressors may cause your ADHD symptoms to increase exponentially. With the whirlwind of demands, this is the time when you're most likely to search for help if you've not yet been formally diagnosed with ADHD.

As you become more comfortable in your relationship and the intensity wanes, it can be harder to connect with your partner. You may be thinking about a work project or distracted by the constant demands of young children. Suddenly, your partner becomes an annoyance. He forgets to close the toilet lid, and in your overreactive state, you take it to mean that he doesn't really care about you. Innocent personal comments can be taken as harsh criticisms and can hack away at your sensitive core, causing you to lash out or withdraw.

Handling Conflict: Fight or Flight?

Did you know that arguing can be a source of stimulation that your brain craves or that you might pick a fight because you're bored or want to release pent-up energy? Many women with ADHD get hooked on excessive exercise, video games, computer activities, or overeating as a manifestation of seeking out stimuli. Who, then, is a more convenient target for your frustration than the person you see day in and day out? Does your partner ever make comments or ask questions like these?

- Why do you have to disagree with everything I say?

- You're just trying to pick a fight.

- Leave me alone!

- I'm just trying to help. Quit picking on me.

If so, maybe it's time to ask yourself if there is a part of you that *likes* the excitement of a good fight. Or, if you are the inattentive subtype, perhaps instead of starting a fight, you obsess, withdraw, or create mountains out of molehills, behaviors that still result in unnecessary conflict. Either way, if you don't redirect this behavior early on, it can become ingrained in your relationship.

When Sex Hurts

Tactile defensiveness (hypersensitivity to touch) often plays a huge part in making intimate moments difficult. Perhaps you've been able to fake it or bite the bullet in the early stages, but now you're facing a lifetime together. You can't fake it forever.

Just as many hyperactive/impulsive women might crave intense physical contact to calm down their nervous system, if you are tactilely defensive, you might find sex to be downright uncomfortable, if not painful. You might flinch if your partner touches you too roughly or, conversely, too lightly. You may retract and ultimately want to avoid sex altogether. All these years, you might have thought you were the odd one out, but I can tell you that the situations described above are quite common. Such intimacy issues can be very troubling, even for couples who are truly committed for the long haul.

Stage 4: Mature Love

By now, you and your partner are comfortable with each other and have fallen into well-established routines. However, after years of trying to manage it all, it may finally be catching up with you. Feelings of exhaustion, being overwhelmed, frustration, or depression often come along with the shift in hormones related to perimenopause or menopause. You might also be tempted to stray due to the boredom of routine. By now, you may also have hit your partner's resentment threshold. Your partner may be "fed up" and want out.

For many, cognitive issues get worse with middle age because of perimenopause or menopause. Attention wanes along with focus and memory, not to mention the drop in libido. This can be a double whammy for a woman with ADHD when it comes to sex. Either she looks for more stimulation and variety to beat the boredom, or she wants to run and hide whenever her partner tries to initiate sex.

Your body is changing now. Maybe you're dealing with weight gain as well as the effects of gravity on your body. You may not feel as physically attractive as you once did. Old self-esteem issues from your teen years about your appearance and desirability may also come up for you.

Not all relationships are weighed down so heavily by a woman's ADHD. In fact, your ever-present creativity and spontaneity can add spice to an otherwise dull, predictable marriage. A partner who is even-keeled and calm may celebrate his wife's colorful personality.

Understanding your ADHD, getting professional help for it (like couples therapy with a therapist who has a strong understanding of ADHD), and learning strategies for managing it can turn your relationship around. Let's look at some solutions for each of the stages to help you do just that.

Stage 1 Solutions: Getting to Know You

The excitement of starting a new love relationship stirs up the ADHD brain, offering it the stimulation it craves, much like a cup of coffee wakes up your morning brain but multiplied by ten thousand. When love, like a superjolt of caffeine, practically lifts you into the air, how do you stay grounded and safe? How do you keep your focus? Above all, whether you're hyperactive/impulsive or inattentive (or a combination of both), it is imperative that you get the appropriate treatment to manage your ADHD *before* getting into a relationship. Assuming that you are already getting help, below are suggestions for managing your ADHD brain as it falls in love.

"Sit, Libido, Sit!"

If your impulsivity contributes to making poor, dangerous decisions, think ahead and come up with alternatives. If you know you're likely to go home with a stranger you've just met at a nightclub, stop going to nightclubs, especially if drinking is involved! Or go with a friend who is depending on you for a ride home. Even better, go out as part of a larger group in order to make one-on-one connecting more difficult, especially if a close friend understands your impulsive ways and can intervene. *Try* to avoid heading out where your impulsivity could endanger you. Instead, wait to make healthy one-on-one connections in settings that are safe and that let you actually converse with a potential date, such as a small party with friends or a group meeting based around your interests, such as photography. Impulsivity can also be controlled by ADHD medications, so having a frank discussion with your doctor should help tame your behaviors. This will allow you to think first before acting, often curtailing dangerous, impulsive behavior.

Take Charge of Your Environment

Meeting new people can be excruciating for the inattentive, quiet subtype. Nightclubs and bars and other noisy places might be too intense for you. Look for quiet settings with fewer people so you can more easily interact with others. Join clubs and attend functions that speak to your interests. If you're overly self-conscious, be sure to ask questions of the people you meet. This puts the focus on the other person, and most people like to talk about themselves—it makes them feel special and appreciated. Rely on friends and relatives to set you up with people they think might be a good match for you.

Let's say you've successfully navigated stage 1, and now you've found someone! As your relationship moves toward becoming serious, how do you make it work when your ADHD is there, waiting to trip you up?

Stage 2 Solutions: Getting Serious

There's nothing more exciting than diving into a relationship that seems to be working. The intensity of love, the newness of it, is literally a stimulant in and of itself. Focusing can come more easily for you because everything about you as a couple is novel and new.

Okay, Honey, I'm Listening

There's no question about it: good communication is the foundation of a strong and healthy relationship. Yes, if you have ADHD, it's going to be more work. The outcome of your efforts, however, will be worth it in the long run; you will have started a habit of keeping the lines open to address both your needs and those of your partner.

Managing distractions in a new relationship can be a challenge, especially when communicating. Since many women with ADHD are highly visual, sit in such a way that you can watch your partner's mouth, following his words and also looking into his eyes. These visual "magnets" or cues can help you stay connected.

Your feelings, especially during these early years of the relationship, can get pretty intense, and that intensity can become overwhelming at times. If you are a highly internal, inattentive subtype, it's likely that you are constantly reacting and feeling very deeply. In order to protect yourself from being overwhelmed, try repeating your parnter's words in your head, putting yourself in his shoes. For example, if he says something totally benign such as "You're having a tough time deciding what to order from the menu," you might immediately begin to ruminate or feel shame because you've been distracted by the chatter at the next table. Instead of taking it as a personal criticism, imagine to yourself what his experience is at that moment: he's simply noticing that you haven't ordered. There is no judgment being placed on you. He's just making an observation and maybe even a kind offer to help. Putting yourself in his place will take you out of your own head and help you stay in the moment. Also, the extra stimulus of touch, such as holding your partner's hand when you talk, can help keep you in the here and now.

A lot of partners of those with ADHD complain that their partners ramble and/or jump to the next thought without a clear path of connection, especially when they discuss an emotionally laden topic. This makes it hard for the partner to follow the conversation. In her book *What Does Everybody Else Know That I Don't?* (1999, 144), Michele Novotni, PhD, points out that many people with ADHD change the topic of conversation frequently. You may see a connection between two subjects, but your listener might not and will get completely lost. Novotni suggests you "pull a conversation back by explaining the links in your own mind. So if you find yourself going off on what appear to others as tangents, be sure to explain how the thoughts are connected in your mind. This will help others view you as a good listener."

When you feel flooded with emotion, your brain doesn't function optimally, and it can be quite difficult to think clearly, making it hard to hold your own end of the conversation. When you're preparing to enter into a serious conversation with your partner, write down the most important points you want to share. This will help solidify and clarify your thinking. If your conversation is spontaneous, and you didn't have time to prepare, instead of running out of the room or shutting down, try drawing on these phrases: "What I'm really trying to say is…" and "The most important thing I want you to understand is…"

Paraphrasing out loud can also help you stay connected and tame your impatience. At a minimum, you can repeat your partner's words in your own head. Another trick is to practice deep breathing to calm yourself while listening and to focus your attention on a part of your body, such as your hands. This brings you into your body and helps you stay present.

If you often find yourself taking over the conversation, a common occurrence with impulsivity, you will need to learn the dance of communicating so that there is a balance—a give-and-take—in your communication. Try this: time yourself while speaking for a minute or two and then pause to give the other person a chance to jump in. Count to three in your head or subtly tap a fingertip to the tip of your thumb three times. Novotni (1999) suggests learning from others by eavesdropping at a mall or other public place and observing the way people talk to each other, pausing and nodding and allowing the conversation to flow seamlessly.

One of the most difficult things to do in any new relationship is to disclose personal information that is important for the other person to know. In this case, it's your ADHD. Do you tell? How? When?

When Do You Disclose ADHD in a Relationship?

What should you say and how much should you reveal? My suggestion is to reveal your ADHD in degrees, depending upon the level of commitment in your relationship.

Keeping It Light

In the early stage of your relationship, in which you are just getting to know each other, there's no need to go over the top with self-disclosure. Too much information (TMI) can scare a person away, and many with ADHD do have an impulsive tendency to talk too much about very personal things. It's best to start light, using descriptors instead of throwing your diagnosis on the table. For example, "I struggle with organization and getting to places on time. And sometimes, I'm forgetful. What's your name again? Ha, ha." As things become more serious, it's time to be more open about your personal issues, just as it is for your partner.

Moving Toward Commitment

If your relationship progresses, and you both want to make a deeper commitment to each other, this is a time in which you and your partner may open up and discuss your vulnerabilities, secrets, and anything that you need to "put on the table" in order for the relationship to move forward in an honest, loving way. To start, explain that the behaviors you described before are symptoms of ADHD and that you have been diagnosed with it. Don't make it sound like a death sentence, because it isn't, but do be clear that your symptoms affect you and might possibly affect him. It is imperative that he understand what ADHD is and how you manage it, and it's just as important for him to know that you are getting help for it or that it is well controlled (if it is!). Since you are getting serious, you also need to let him know that ADHD is a genetic disorder. Remember the 1996 study by Biederman and colleagues that states that "strongly increased risks for ADHD (57%) among the offspring of adults with ADHD have been reported." It's only fair to share this information up front.

Now remember, *everyone* has issues, and though your ADHD may seem huge to you, it might not be that big of a problem for your partner. You want to share both your challenges *and* your strengths as a unique individual as well as a woman who happens to have ADHD. Your ADHD doesn't define you. It's only part of who you are. Certainly, your new love has foibles, too. Perhaps bring that out in the discussion as well, in a kind but playful way: "You mentioned that you suck at sports. Well, I suck at folding clothes."

Okay, Buster, You Need to Understand Me

If you are now in a long-term committed relationship, but your partner doesn't take you seriously, doesn't believe ADHD exists, or takes your behavior personally, then educate him about ADHD. Ask him to read the excellent book *Driven to Distraction* by Drs. Hallowell and Ratey. Invite him to local support groups. CHADD (Children and Adults with ADHD) has local chapters in most large cities (1-800-233-4050, http://www.chadd.org).

Take advantage of this romantic stage of your relationship to ask your partner to take some time to get to know you even more deeply. Now that you've been together and settled into a serious partnership, hopefully your partner has a solid understanding of ADHD and how it affects you, him, your relationship, and your family and friends.

Stage 3 Solutions: The Honeymoon Is Over

As lovebirds turn into partners with a deep commitment to each other, your relationship changes yet again. Now that you're formally a team and know each other quite well, you both are seeing how your ADHD affects you as a couple and as a family.

The Importance of a Positive ADD-itude

You cannot allow your partner to complain or criticize your ADHD-related behaviors any more than if you had a hearing impairment and needed him to speak more loudly and clearly. In a healthy, loving relationship, you support each other's needs with empathy and kindness. ADHD doesn't go away and there is no cure. But by getting the help you need to manage your symptoms so that they don't get in the way, you are showing him (and you!) that you can take some control over the situation.

From the beginning, explain the difference between enabling and support. You may need to keep repeating this over the first few years of your relationship until your partner really gets it. Enabling is treating you like a helpless child. You aren't helpless. You are a competent adult who needs a helping hand now and then. It's important to get his support and have him on board without him being condescending, taking on a parental role, or otherwise undermining you as an intelligent, healthy, independent adult. Explain why you need outside help around the house, like a cleaning crew. If he doesn't have time or otherwise isn't able to pitch in, hiring cleaning help is no more of a luxury than getting hearing aids would be. Certainly there are times when your partner needs *your* help. When you *gently* point out the differences between enabling and support, this will help him to "get" you, especially if you've never taught him what living with ADHD is all about. Ask him to focus on your strengths more than on your challenges, just as he would want you to do for him. It's certainly not the end of the world to have ADHD, and with treatment and a kind, supportive partner, the positives will far outweigh the negatives.

When ADHD Follows You into the Bedroom

First, read as much as possible about ADHD and relationships to better understand how your ADHD interferes with intimacy. (See http://ADDconsults.com for a list of books on this subject.) Chances are your difficulties have been chronic, and neither you nor your partner ever understood the connection. With understanding comes the ability to solve problems.

Take Action Against Distraction

If distractibility is an issue, there are a number of things you can do to help you stay focused. Start with the basics:

- Since your medication has most likely worn off by late evening, your symptoms might be raging. If that interferes with intimacy, discuss medication tweaking with your physician. Adding an extra dose or taking your meds later in the day might help. (Important: Do *not* make medication changes without first discussing them with your health care provider.)

- If boredom is the issue, talk with your partner about ways to make sex more exciting. Try new positions or locations (private, of course) and read books or go online for tips.

- Turn off all distractions: TV, lights (though for some, seeing more instead of less is helpful), and phones.

- Set up romance dates in advance to help you get in the mood. Many women have complained that a spontaneous suggestion from a mate is too difficult due to their ADHD difficulties with transitions. Ask your partner to schedule time or give you plenty of hints and lots of time to shift your attention.

- Take regular romantic getaways where your focus is on each other. If you have kids, ask family or friends to take them so you have total privacy. Even if it's a short weekend now and again, it's important to find the time to stay connected.

- Talk about what you're feeling and experiencing during lovemaking as a way to stay connected and focused (as long as that doesn't make you even more distracted). Look deeply into each other's eyes to increase those feelings of connection.

Talk About Touch

What feels good for one woman with ADHD may feel completely different for another woman with ADHD. Again, open discussions with your partner are necessary. Don't expect your partner to be a mind reader. Explain and demonstrate what feels good and what doesn't. Some women with ADHD find that sex calms down their nervous systems by virtue of the heaviness of their partner's body. Many women have told me that their hyperactive/impulsive body craves that type of sensory experience and that the sexual act itself is often secondary. This is akin to the calming effect of sleeping under heavy blankets. A hyperactive woman might find sexual activity pleasurable because of the intense physical contact—the thrill of the moment—and the disinhibited physical movement involved. The hypersensitive, inattentive woman may require a lot of time to "warm up" and may be especially particular about how she is touched. Regardless of your subtype, clear but loving communication is needed to make your lovemaking pleasurable for both of you. Intimacy takes many forms, physical and emotional. Having a solid relationship requires good communication skills in general. The communication skills you practice when talking about sensitive issues such as sex can also serve you well when you and your partner confront conflict.

Conflict Can Be Productive, but Harmony Is Even Better

As life becomes more complicated, so does your relationship with your partner. There is so much going on, and your ADHD can, and often will, get in the way, causing tension between you. The first thing you can do is take preventative measures to manage your stress in order to reduce your symptoms, which in turn will help reduce conflict, especially if you tend to pick a fight just to blow off some steam. Here are a few reminders:

- Identify the stressors. Is it keeping up with household chores? Managing the kids? Hire help (cleaning service/babysitters) whenever you are in stress overload. If cost is an issue, barter with friends or neighbors.

- Exercise, exercise, exercise! This has proved to be great medicine for ADHD.

- Nurture yourself with hobbies, time with friends, hot baths—whatever rings your bell.

- Get adequate sleep and good nutrition.

Once your nervous system is in good shape, you'll be in a much better position to resolve conflict more productively. For the inattentive woman, here are some tips to make this work for you.

Inattentives, Take the Bull by the Horns!

If you're the inattentive subtype, you are more likely to avoid conflict altogether. This only fuels your anger and your partner's resentment. To avoid the flooding of emotions, loss of words, and being unable to hold your ground when entering into conflict, try staying in the present. Breathe deeply to help calm yourself down. If you know ahead of time that you will be having an unsettling discussion with your partner, practice saying what's on your mind to give you some confidence. Try presenting your complaints as problems that need to be solved rather than finger pointing and accusing, which will only make your partner become defensive, escalating into anger and worse. If need be, remove yourself from the situation until you can settle down, then return and calmly hold your ground until you get your message across. Remember to give and take, listen and talk, and, when possible, use "I" messages, such as "I feel like you don't care about my feelings when you make sarcastic comments about…" It's easy to get so caught up in conflict that your chronic insecurities return, making you feel vulnerable and angry, resulting in overreactivity.

How to Keep the Pot from Boiling Over

After you and your partner have been together for a while, you come to know each other's hot spots. Even a hint of criticism can unleash a reactive hurling of angry words. If he pleads innocence and criticizes you for being "oversensitive," calmly explain that your sensitivities are brain based, very real, and part of your ADHD. Describe areas of *good* hypersensitivities, such as how you care deeply about other people, the state of the world, ecology, and other issues, so he can place your sensitivities on a continuum. Gently point out how certain triggers take you down and how they impact your relationship. Give him examples of how best to talk to you about his frustrations to avoid triggering you. If criticisms that come out of the blue derail you, ask him to set up a time to discuss what is bothering him so you have time to prepare emotionally. Sometimes, when things get terribly heated, it works to e-mail each other. This gives you time to reflect and put your feelings and thoughts into words that might otherwise get tangled up in raw emotion.

In addition to conflict with your partner, you may also experience conflict with the rest of the family. Problems arise—that's just the nature of families—so plan weekly or monthly family meetings. Set the tone by talking about the positives of each person. For example, "It was very thoughtful of you to change the lightbulbs without being asked. I really appreciated that." Then move on to the problem—again stating it as just that, a problem——and ask for ideas on how to solve it. Developing good communication skills takes lots of practice, but in the long run, those skills will enable you to work out areas of conflict with a minimum of hurt feelings. These skills can be learned early on in your relationship and see you through many long years together. However, just when you think you've got the art of relationship down, things change again.

Stage 4 Solutions: Mature Love

At this point, you have become comfortable with each other and you want to leverage your comfort to grow even closer rather than just get stuck in a rut. Some impulsive/hyperactive women may be tempted to "explore" outside of their marriage to alleviate their boredom. If you're inattentive, you might be completely bored with the old routine but have no idea how to fix things, so you just mentally check out. Aside from regular getaways to rekindle your flame, try doing something altogether different to change the routine. Take dance lessons. If you watch TV every night, try doing something different: go miniature golfing or explore new activities you both might enjoy. Invite friends over or meet up at a restaurant or movie. To keep your relationship rich, do the unexpected: leave little love notes where he can find them. In *A.D.D. & Romance* (1998), Jonathan Scott Halverstadt, MS, suggests using your ADHD symptoms, such as impulsivity, to enrich your relationship. In one example, he describes a time when he stopped at a store to buy some medicine and noticed a teddy bear. Knowing that his wife passionately collects them, he grabbed one, along with a bunch of her favorite flowers, red carnations. Surprise can go a long way to inject some positive energy! We also often forget to compliment those we've lived with for so long—instead, we point out faults—so find a way to compliment him about something every day.

360-Degree-Acceptance

One of the benefits of aging is the opportunity to experience life through the lens of acceptance. This means learning to accept not only your partner's foibles, but also your own. This acceptance may involve forgiving yourself for things you can't change and working to change those things that you can.

Practice seeing yourself as someone who is capable and has gifts and strengths. We all do, but they can be hard to accept if your focus is constantly on your weaknesses. Sometimes it helps to be concrete—say, by writing down all the things that are going *right* instead of hyperfocusing on what is going wrong. Make a list of your assets, your strengths. Think of what people have said to you, whether it's that you're a good listener, a great baker, a good singer, a gifted attorney, or whatever. If you're having difficulties with this, then it might be time to work with a therapist—preferably one with experience working with adults who have ADHD—to sort things out.

Now that you've worked on acceptance, what's next? It's time to turn our attention to...inattention.

Tuning Back In

Inattention is a huge problem within couples' relationships, especially when, after being together for years, you think you've heard it all a thousand times before. This is the most important person in your life and you need to hear what he is saying. Remind yourself that you really need to pay attention when he is talking to you—no easy feat! Get into the habit of stopping what you are doing. STOP, DROP (what you're doing), and really LISTEN. If you're a slow processor—another common ADHD trait that has nothing to do with intelligence—ask him to slow down. Again, repeat in your head what you just heard. Sometimes it helps to even repeat it out loud.

Rheumatoid Romance

Despite some women's wandering eyes and/or loss of interest in sex in the later years of a relationship, on the positive side, once any kids you have are gone, this can be a time to relax your inhibitions and really explore. It's an opportunity to develop more mature, loving expressions that are less about performance and more about genuine connection. At this point, you may find freedom in having a greater acceptance of each other. You can enjoy your comfort level.

On the other hand, if you are the hyperactive, impulsive subtype, you may find yourself tempted to start an affair. Do some deep reflection before acting on your impulses if you're thinking about this. How will it make you feel in the long run? How would you feel if it were the other way around? Imagine the repercussions if your partner finds out. Talk it out with a trusted friend. This temptation is also a signal that something is very wrong with your relationship and needs immediate attention. This could be a wake-up call. If you act out your fantasies, you can't take it back. It's less the act itself in most cases than the deceit and the loss of trust that damage a relationship.

Instead of putting that energy into an extramarital affair, you can choose to put it into the relationship that you now have. If you are a mom who is now an "empty nester," you can enjoy your marriage in a new, fresh way now that the kids are older. You have a choice: you can use that energy for something that may be terribly hurtful to the one you love or to enhance your partnership.

Here are a few ideas to spark your relationship: How about starting a business together? Or taking a long, adventurous trip together, something you've always wanted to do, like walking *El Camino de Santiago* in Spain or taking a cruise through the Inside Passage in Alaska? Or joining the Peace Corps or volunteering together for Habitat for Humanity? Or perhaps moving to a different state? Any one of these could shake things up and enliven your relationship. But if you're at the point of actually acting out your impulse to stray, it's imperative to get to a therapist to sort things out.

Despite all the challenges of having ADHD and being in a relationship, there can also be much joy, pleasure, and companionship. Your partner is a person you can now trust with all the secret feelings you brought in from your youth. This is one of the few relationships in which you can truly be yourself, and, hopefully, be accepted and cherished for your authentic self.

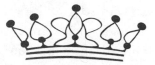

CHAPTER 8

So I'm Sensitive. Sue Me!

Cindy and Amanda, both in their early forties and friends since childhood, hadn't seen each other in nearly twenty years. Amanda had moved over one thousand miles away after graduating from college. When she returned for a visit, she and Cindy met up at a restaurant that had recently opened in their old hometown. As soon as they sat down, Cindy, who has inattentive ADHD, started feeling ill. The place was packed. Music blared in the background, ceiling fans whirred in her line of vision, and the hubbub of chatter filled the air. As excited as she was to see her old friend, Cindy quickly began to feel queasy and anxious. Amanda commented how much she loved the restaurant. She became more energized as she raised her voice in order to be heard over the din. Cindy began to shut down, afraid she was going to pass out, and felt a panic attack coming on, something she'd experienced many times before when feeling overwhelmed. Though Amanda never even noticed, Cindy's feelings of being overwhelmed prevented her from enjoying the outing with her oldest friend. She barely heard a word that was spoken.

Like Cindy, many women with ADHD live with extreme sensitivity to sight, sound, smell, taste, and touch. This high level of sensitivity to stimuli can be overwhelming for them in a number of situations that are humdrum for other people. Their ADHD brains are not able to "tune out" input, so these women experience it as a painful barrage of stimuli coming at them all at once. Going to the mall can feel like being in a nightmarish carnival fun house. Large parties, loud restaurants with blaring music and TVs, the cleaning products aisle in the grocery store, or wearing itchy, binding clothing are all examples of situations that can increase the stress levels of women with ADHD to the point where it interferes with their already compromised ability to concentrate or focus.

Women with ADHD are either attracted to stimuli or repelled by them. It's often one extreme or the other, with the inattentive woman craving quiet and the hyperactive woman seeking lights, camera, ACTION! Though there are times when the inattentive woman also seeks out stimulating experiences, which often "brings her up to normal," and the hyperactive woman looks for downtime to restore her energy level, it's often the case that the inattentive woman seeks quiet experiences where she can reflect internally, whereas the hyperactive woman expresses her needs more externally.

Overly stimulating situations can increase the attention and focus of the hyperactive woman, whereas the same environment can distract, overwhelm, and shut down the inattentive woman. Places like Disneyland, Vegas, sporting events, or even shopping malls can be compelling and pleasurable settings for the hyperactive woman, whereas the inattentive woman might prefer to seek out a quiet reading spot by the lake where she can sit for hours, lost in her own world.

NOISE!

Many inattentive women seem to hear sounds that no one else notices. In fact, my own ADHD diagnosis came about because I thought I was losing my hearing. When I was on the telephone, I couldn't hear the person on the other end if there was even the slightest sound in the room, like a quiet TV or a family member talking. I couldn't even filter out the gentle whoosh of the air vent fan! A hearing test confirmed that there was no problem with my ears. In fact, my hearing was more acute than that of most my age. I didn't realize at the time that I simply could not filter out extraneous sounds; nor could I pick out one voice from a small group. To this day, I always put a finger in my free ear while I'm talking on the phone—even in an empty room.

As you can see in Cindy and Amanda's story above, noise is one of the major areas of sensory sensitivity. Though both hyperactive/impulsive and inattentive women can be supersensitive to stimulation, inattentive women are most likely to have a heightened sensory experience, whereas hyperactive women are often (but not always) too distracted to notice. Women with ADHD, regardless of subtype, may find it hard to deal with places that have a lot of stimuli, such as conversations (for example, at parties, events, or meetings), loud music, hustle and bustle, loud fans, kitchen-related noise, TVs, and radios.

Though an exaggerated startle response to sudden noise has not been documented in the research on ADHD, many women with ADHD have it—the experience is commonly reported to clinicians. It's not uncommon that a woman with ADHD will jump a foot out of her chair at the sound of fireworks, balloons popping, gunshots, or a sudden shriek or unexpected peal of loud laughter. Traffic sounds, like trucks, motorcycles, and bad exhaust pipes, can make a woman with ADHD feel like she's in the middle of a combat zone. Her fight-or-flight response kicks in immediately, often triggering anxiety or even a mini panic attack.

Even relaxing outside in your own backyard no longer offers opportunities to tune out and calm down when the neighborhood is full of the sounds of lawn mowing, hedge trimming, drilling, cars roaring down the street, and kids squealing in swimming pools.

Indoors is no better as you try to shut out the noises of electrical appliances (including those that no one else seems to be able to hear), such as the humming of fluorescent lights, the fridge, the air conditioner, TVs, radios, computers, and garbage disposals, as well as the sounds of people chewing food and making other "mouth" noises. And the worst offender of all (at least for me) is the vacuum cleaner. This reaction to noise even follows you to work, where you may be bombarded by the sounds of telephones, copy machines, coworkers' conversations, and more. Let's face it—noise is everywhere.

The Skin You're In

Your skin is your largest organ. You might find that contact with certain textures or even a gentle hug can push someone with your sensitivity right over the top.

Clothing: Can't Live With It, Can't Live Without It

Suffice it to say that this is one of the most troubling areas of sensitivity for women because it's something you cannot escape unless you live in a nudist colony. You can avoid crowded, noisy restaurants or parties. You can change the lightbulbs in your house from fluorescent to incandescent. You can buy white-noise machines and sleep masks to help you sleep. But you cannot avoid wearing clothes. Hopefully, the pointers offered in chapter 5 will assist you in finding a happy middle ground—rather than getting arrested for indecent exposure!

Intimate Touch: The Agony or the Ecstasy?

Even pleasurable skin contact can be problematic for women hypersensitive to touch. Hugs from loved ones can be torturous because of neurological sensitivity. Light stroking, enjoyed by most, can result in painful tickling sensations. Foreplay and intercourse can also be unpleasant and even painful.

Satin Sheets Are a Girl's Best Friend

When it comes to bedding, the Princess and the Pea syndrome once again follows the woman with ADHD into the bedroom. Many have to make their beds *before* retiring for sleep, making sure that every wrinkle is removed, so that they can sleep without being distracted by their bodies sweeping over the creases. Though some prefer the least amount of bedding on them as possible (the weight can feel too restricting), many find the opposite to be true. I've heard from numerous women with ADHD that the pressure and weight of heavy blankets and comforters can have a calming effect and are often used even in the heat of summer. My own daughter, who has ADHD, wears two layers of pajamas and finds that using several heavy blankets helps her fall asleep.

Gooey, Gunky, Icky, Sticky Substances

I have heard hundreds of women with ADHD over the years complain about their sensitivity to sticky, gooey stuff. For some reason, this particular sensation is especially disturbing for those with ADHD. For a woman with extreme sensory sensitivities, touching a gooey cabinet knob can have the same effect as fingernails on a blackboard might for the person without ADHD. It can cause an immediate aversion and feeling of repulsion. I once worked with a woman with ADHD who described sticky floors as the worst sensory nightmare she could think of. With two young children at home, she felt disgust every time she had to touch a doorknob or pull a cabinet or refrigerator handle covered in jelly, juice, or some other sticky substance. In fact, she recalled how even as a four-year-old in preschool she refused to touch finger paints, looking on in bewilderment as her classmates enthusiastically dunked their hands in the goop and smeared it around on large sheets of paper. Another woman explained it this way: "People might think I have OCD or am a cleaning nut because I spend so much time wiping counters, doorknobs, and floors, but the truth is, the sensation of stickiness on my hands or feet sends me right over the edge." These women are not alone. Their hypersensitivity to sticky, gooey substances that cause quite a bit of distress is shared by others with ADHD; many even feel repulsion at putting on sunscreen or makeup.

In the Eye of the Beholder

Though not discussed as much as other types of sensory input that can become overwhelming to women with ADHD, visual stimuli are often problematic as well. Monica, a woman who attended my ADD support group, was particularly reactive to lighting. She felt queasy in rooms with fluorescent lights; therefore, many shopping experiences made her feel so ill that she left as soon as she could. She often felt uncomfortable in movie theaters because the screen encompassed her entire field of vision, making her feel claustrophobic and overwhelmed (a sensation not helped by the increased volume and the quick cuts from one shot to another in rapid-fire movements). She avoided restaurants that had multiple TVs and ceiling fans, because the movement of the images onscreen and the fan blades would send her into dizzy spells. Grocery shopping was torturous, as the shelves screamed out to her with their multiple patterns and colors at every turn. At restaurants, she chose her table carefully, avoiding windows that might bounce off glare into her sensitive eyes, preferring a booth against a wall instead. Patterned or striped wallpaper and checkerboard floors made her lose her appetite. It all overwhelmed her senses! Even reading could be problematic: newspapers, magazines, and books often had too much text, or the text was too small, so she preferred large-print literature sprinkled with lots of white space or graphics.

Scent-sitivity

The amount of scented products on the market is staggering. Thanks to marketing strategies, we're brainwashed to think that natural (and usually perfectly acceptable) odors must be covered up: there are sprays and scented candles to freshen the air, perfumes to attract the opposite sex and make women seem more desirable, deodorants and soaps filled with perfumes to prevent body odor, detergents and dryer sheets to make laundry smell better than fresh. These artificial scents can take a toll on women with extreme sense-sitivities, often sending them into bronchial spasms or migraines.

The other extreme is the reaction to everyday smells that others may be able to tolerate more easily: certain foods can trigger a gag response. One woman I worked with felt sick to her stomach whenever she awoke to the smell of bacon wafting through the air. It was simply too early for her senses to experience such a jarring, strong smell, even one that most find extremely appealing. Body odors, though unpleasant to many, can send a woman with ADHD reaching for her scarf or tissue to block out the offending smell, especially if she's stuck in the subway, on a bus, or in a checkout line.

Empathy, Sympathy, and Overreactivity

Though it is not considered one of the five senses, many women with ADHD often have heightened emotional sensitivity as well. Criticism, for example, may feel like a direct attack on your very being, often causing an immediate breakdown of self-esteem. Part of this reaction, often going back to early childhood, may be due to many years of hearing criticism for being late, being messy, not finishing projects, and so on. Years later, these continue to be triggers that attack the core of your self-worth, and you then react either by blowing up, running away, or freezing, feeling too overwhelmed with intense feelings to be able to hold your ground in an argument. Quite often you internalize the criticism, which, in turn, can lead to depression. Best-selling author and ADHD expert Sari Solden (2005, 87, 89) writes eloquently about the emotional journey of living with ADHD in her book *Women with Attention Deficit Disorder: Embrace Your Differences and Transform Your Life*. As Solden says, "It's easy to understand...why a woman would be reactive. I conceive of it as if these women start out each day with ninety percent of their coping vessel already filled. Combine this with chaos, disorganization, and the energy it takes to cope each day, and we can see why it wouldn't take much to put someone over the top." She goes on to say that "being overwhelmed, overloaded, and overworked, being nonassertive, engaging in negative self-talk, and being highly reactive with quickly changing moods can all leave women locked in a state of depression."

This hypersensitivity (and the tears that often follow) can be set off by a wide array of everyday external triggers ranging from something as simple as a sappy commercial to movies, music, and art. It is not uncommon for a woman with ADHD also to feel intense reactions (more than average) to major life events and transitions like births, deaths, or children starting kindergarten or graduating from college.

The woman with ADHD is often even more susceptible to "overfeeling" when she is premenstrual. These difficulties either worsen or improve with menopause. Dr. Patricia Quinn (2002, 87, 99), who has done extensive work in the field of ADHD and women's hormones, writes, "Treatment regimes [sic] [for women with ADHD] are usually made up of recommendations established from the experience of treating elementary school–aged boys. Hormonal fluctuations and the influences of estrogen on the brain are not even considered, much less addressed." She adds that "the key to better outcomes for women with ADHD lies not only in better recognition of the disorder, but in the realization that, in addition to their ADHD, these women must cope with an ever-changing hormonal environment that can have a significant impact on ADHD and coexisting symptoms."

Many women with ADHD have an overly developed sense of empathy and tend to be highly tuned into and responsive to the emotional states of others. On the other hand, some women with ADHD might seem to *lack* empathy toward others' feelings and points of view, but often this latter group of women is simply too distracted to notice others' feelings. (See chapter 7, on relationships.)

And finally, these intense internal feelings can almost have the quality of OCD (obsessive-compulsive disorder) as women ruminate endlessly over past events, feelings, and perceived "screw-ups." These are women who are often criticized unfairly for "thinking too much, too hard" and being "too sensitive."

Supports for the Sensory Sensitive Soul

As we consider the sensitivities discussed earlier, let's look at some simple solutions to help manage the stress of being overwhelmed. For example, when going out to eat, the woman with ADHD should choose the restaurant and the table whenever possible so as to minimize distractions. When it comes to clothing, she can order special clothing online or from catalogs made with fabrics that are designed to be easy on ultrasensitive skin. And ordering online or from catalogs means she doesn't have to face the mall! She can change the lighting in her workplace and in her home to reduce glare, and she can replace all of her home and body products with unscented, all natural ones. These are just a few of the many excellent suggestions in this chapter to help make the world feel like a more welcoming place. There is no reason you have to go through the rest of your life feeling uncomfortable in your own skin. A few simple adjustments here and there can make all the difference. Life is too short to spend it being uncomfortable! Now let's look at some more solutions for sensory sensitivities.

Hey, World, Can Ya Turn Down the Volume, Please?

It's impossible to avoid noise—it's everywhere—but there are ways to minimize its effects. When shopping, for example, go to smaller stores and boutiques whenever possible, or better yet, purchase your items via catalogs or online stores. If you absolutely must head to the mall, wear earplugs or headphones playing soft, gentle music. In restaurants, find the quietest booth or table. You can even ask the host or hostess for this consideration, as he or she often knows the quieter spots. Traditionally, many women follow societal norms and find it difficult to express their needs, suppressing them in favor of keeping the peace or putting others' needs first. With practice, you can learn to speak up and become more self-confident while maintaining consideration of others' needs at the same time. This is the first step in learning to advocate for yourself and your needs. If the host or hostess at a restaurant leads you to a table in the middle of a children's birthday party, speak up as soon as possible and politely request a quieter location!

Social outings and gatherings can be disastrous because of your inability to hear over even the slightest noise. One way to get around this is to say to your companions that you'd really like to hear what they have to say and that you'd rather be in a place where you can give them your full attention.

Other Tips for Dealing with Being Overwhelmed by Noise

There's no reason to be a prisoner of your hypersensitivity to sound. Take charge and try these tips:

- If you can't get out of a situation, take frequent sensory-free breaks.

- If you know you're going to be miserable at a certain location, suggest another meeting place, vacation spot, or whatever.

- Avoid loud, noisy situations whenever possible. This is about self-care. If you know you're going to be miserable, it's okay to say no even if "everyone else is going." At a big party, seek out one or two people and find a quieter spot off to a corner, in another room, or outside.

- White noise, fans, and nature sounds (use a laptop and find looping channels or download pleasant audio files to your iPod) work great in noisy hotels, office settings, and similar situations.

- Bring your iPhone or iPod loaded with gentle music to the movies for emergency relief—or bring earplugs.

Unpleasant sounds are everywhere, every day. By recognizing which are the most offensive and taking action using the tips and techniques above, you can learn how to live in a loud, chaotic world.

How to Turn Your Sensual Sensitivity into a Win-Win

Hang in there, ladies! There are numerous ways to turn sensual, sexual intimacy from discomfort to joy. Open, honest communication with your partner is essential. Educate him as to your overall sensitivities so he understands that there is a larger context, not just sex. This will also help your partner not take your reaction personally. Explain what feels good and what doesn't feel good. If a tight hug is too confining, suggest other options. If light touch is too ticklish, ask for a deep massage. While some inattentive women are overwhelmed with the intensity of sexual stimuli and sensation of skin on skin, others (often hyperactive women) find that sexual activity is calming; they crave heaviness and closeness, which, like a heavy blanket or comforter, tends to settle down their hyperactivity. Whatever your subtype or preference, sexual foreplay and intercourse need to be a pleasurable experience for both you and your partner. Guide your lover! No one can read your mind.

Put on Your Rose-Colored Glasses

There are also many ways to work with your visual sensitivities. Make sunglasses your best friend. Just as earplugs muffle annoying sounds, sunglasses will help soften bright light and keep you from being visually overwhelmed. Again, the large screens found at the movie theater may be too powerful for your eyes and other senses. Wait for the movie to come out on cable and enjoy watching it in the comfort of your own home on a smaller screen. If you must head to the movies, sit as far back as possible so you're not pulled into the visual abyss of the screen. Avoid

3-D movies if possible, and sit near the aisle if you need a break requiring a quick exit. Above all, make sure your companion understands your sensitivities ahead of time.

Other Tips for Dealing with Being Overwhelmed Visually

Just as there are ways to muffle overwhelming sounds, there are strategies you can use to "dim the lights" as well. Here are some tips to help tame overwhelming visual stimuli:

- At home, replace all plain fluorescent bulbs with soft, full-spectrum fluorescent lightbulbs.

- Use natural lighting as much as possible, but draw the shades if the sun is too intense or wear sunglasses inside.

- Turn off the overhead lights and use floor and table lamps for a softer mood.

- When eating out, choose a booth or table next to a wall to avoid glare from windows or the sun. Try not to sit in places where you can see fans and TVs, customer foot traffic, and the register.

- When reading, use paper to cover up the parts of the page you're not reading. A ruler works well to keep your vision from jumping around the page. Choose books with lots of white space, and if possible, pick a book that has large print.

- Use e-readers to take advantage of font size options, page colors, and reading formats.

- When shopping, head to smaller stores, preferably freestanding stores rather than malls (which are more likely to have fluorescent rather than natural lighting).

You don't have to be a victim of your overstimulating environment. Take charge and find peace and calm in your otherwise hectic day.

The Sweet Smell of Success

Luckily, many companies are developing more and more "green" products, so it's easier than ever to find things that won't overwhelm your sense of smell. You can now find unscented or natural deodorants, makeup, detergent, and cleaning products. However, some things are still out of your control, so once again, it helps to be proactive in order to protect yourself and stand up for your needs. Learn to use "I" statements. For example, if you know you'll be lunching with a friend who favors perfumes, mention beforehand that though the scent is indeed lovely, you have a severe reaction to heavy scents. Many folks, indeed, do have allergies and chemical sensitivities, so people are generally becoming more understanding of such differences. If you find yourself seated next to someone in public, cornered and overpowered by perfume, remove yourself if possible; explain briefly that you have an allergy to perfume, if it's needed. If moving isn't an option, take your umbrella and club them over the head, then run to the bus driver and ask to be taken off immediately. Kidding!

So I Cry at Movies—Big Deal!

Though "overfeeling" can be distressing at times, there are ways to get through it without denying your sensitive soul. The first step is to understand your ADHD and come to a place of acceptance. Your reactivity, though intense and sometimes embarrassing, is, on the other hand, a wonderful trait because it shows your sensitivity and empathy for others. Celebrate the richness and compassion it brings instead of shuddering in embarrassment. Embrace your kind heart, creativity, and talents. Most creative women feel things very strongly and use their art, music, writing, dance, or form of other creative expression as a way to share these deep inner experiences.

Other Tips for Dealing with Being Overwhelmed Emotionally

Being a sensitive person is nothing to be ashamed of. Below are some tips, though, to help you through the rough spots:

- Find a go-to "safe" person who can offer support during intense moments. Talk things out with that person instead of holding it in.

- Reject toxic help from those who describe you as being "overly" sensitive.

- Use self-talk to calm down and to remind yourself not to take anything personally. Don't make assumptions. Get the facts whenever possible to help avoid emotional meltdowns.

- Take five. When verbal disagreements begin to turn into unhealthy fights and you find yourself unable to hold your ground, remove yourself until you are calm enough to engage in a more productive discussion.

- Use creative or calm ways to express your feelings. Writing is a great tool for releasing emotions, helping you prepare for a difficult conversation, or organizing your thoughts.

- Consider psychotherapy with someone who has experience and expertise in working with people with ADHD to help you sort out feelings and reactions.

These are just a handful of tips to help you during those moments when you are emotionally overwhelmed. Consider other things that have helped you in the past, such as meditation, exercise, or taking a walk, for example. You might also find these two books, which address hypersensitivities in general, helpful: *Too Loud, Too Bright, Too Fast, Too Tight: What to Do If You Are Sensory Defensive in an Overstimulating World* by Sharon Heller, PhD, and *The Highly Sensitive Person* by Elaine Aron, PhD.

Overall Solutions for Hypersensitivities

Being highly sensitive, you may have lived your whole life feeling out of step with the rest of the world, a common reaction to living with ADHD. Inattentive women seem to have the most difficulty. Hyperactive women, on the other hand, might jump into the action but then find that they are totally spent well before the rest because they tend to experience life with incredible intensity. While others are off enjoying roller coasters, scary movies, bustling vacation destinations, and cheerful holiday parties, you may find yourself watching from the wings, feeling left out or even embarrassed.

It's important to reiterate that the hypersensitivities described above are often experienced differently for the hyperactive woman. She may externalize her difficulties through anger or even rage, while the inattentive woman might withdraw into a depression. The hyperactive woman's impulsivity might drive her to do or say things she'll regret later, as she reacts swiftly to being bombarded with stimuli. Whether you're inattentive or hyperactive, it's important to understand your triggers, see them coming, and have a plan so that you can dodge the sensory bullets by being proactive and cutting them off at the pass with your newfound tools and tactics.

Remember, being a sensitive, emotional being is not a bad thing or a weakness. It simply means you feel things more deeply than others. Having an intuitive sense of the world and the people around you helps make you a compassionate person. Being more sensitive than most is like the difference between an orchid and a cactus. Yes, you require more maintenance and careful handling, but you're worth it because you bring the world such exquisite sensitivity.

CHAPTER 9

Hormonal Humps, Bumps, and Flashes

Hey, Girlfriend!

What's up? Hope Max is feeling better. You wouldn't believe the day I'm having. I almost lost my job 'cuz I forgot to hand in my reports (again) and didn't finish that project that was due last week. I have some kind of brain fog, and I'm exhausted all the time. I'm surprised I remember my own name. To make things worse, I can't get this weight off, which is really bringing me down, and my ADD meds may as well be sugar pills. I thought life would be a breeze once the kids left for college and I could focus on me for a change, but instead, it feels like my whole life is falling apart. Sorry for the downer of an update, but I'm barely keeping it together. Hope you are doing okay.

Love,

Rachel

Like a lot of women in midlife, Rachel is perimenopausal—that is, she's in the stage before menopause—but she has not yet made the connection between her worsening ADHD symptoms and her hormonal imbalances. Unfortunately, most women don't put their hormonal changes and the impact on their cognitive functioning together. Take the "normal" hormonal symptoms all women go through in puberty, the fertile years, perimenopause, menopause, and postmenopause, then stir in all the symptoms of ADHD, shake, and you have one killer cocktail. Unfortunately, there is very little in the way of research and/or writing about this topic. But we do know that, though earlier indicators may be apparent in retrospect, puberty is often the time when a girl shows her first signs of ADHD.

Puberty Ain't Always Purty

Girls with ADHD often don't show symptoms until later than their male counterparts. Relatively speaking, they tend to be quiet and well behaved, whereas boys with ADHD are more likely to exhibit behaviors such as hyperactivity and impulsive acting out. If you are a mother with daughters, your girls are statistically at risk for also having ADHD, so it's important to understand how pivotal this time, when her symptoms reveal themselves, may be. Early intervention and treatment are essential before she faces significant difficulties at school, at home, and in social contexts.

During puberty, a girl with ADHD may exhibit various symptoms. She might become more chatty and spacey in school. She may be inattentive in class because she is distracted and finds her inner world much more interesting than the teacher's lectures. As her hormones are changing, and if she's prone to premenstrual syndrome (PMS), she can become more emotionally unstable—more so than a non-ADHD girl entering puberty—with mood swings that can be quite unsettling. She may become more sensitive and reactive, having outbursts at every perceived slight, demand, or criticism. As she moves inward, signs of anxiety and/or depression might reveal themselves. In general, her ADHD symptoms worsen.

It is interesting to note, however, that some symptoms can actually improve. For some girls who are hyperactive and impulsive, the out-of-control hyperactivity seen in earlier childhood subsides with puberty. Instead of the running, swinging off furniture, and such, your daughter might develop restlessness, such as swinging her feet, jiggling her leg, or chattering nonstop. She may also get into team sports, dance, gymnastics, or other physical activities as a more acceptable way to release pent-up energy.

Still, young teens often exhibit major difficulties that need to be recognized and treated. In an article in *ADDitude* magazine (McCarthy 2009), Stephen Hinshaw, PhD, chair of the department of psychology at the University of California, Berkeley, who has been studying girls with ADHD for more than ten years, says, "We found that ADHD girls in their early teens have more academic problems, more aggressive behavior, earlier signs of substance-related problems, and higher rates of depression than girls who don't have the condition." Given the research, if you are a mom, it's important to keep a close eye on your adolescent daughter should she start exhibiting signs of ADHD. If you're not a mom, you might find it interesting to reflect back on your own puberty to recall any early signs of ADHD. In addition to the challenges of puberty, premenstrual syndrome (PMS), which also often starts in puberty, can follow young teens into adulthood, wreaking havoc on women of all ages during their reproductive years.

PMS: Pretty Miserable State

Most women ride "The Wicked Twister," their very own hormonal roller coaster, at times throughout their lives, but the high and lows are even more dramatic when PMS is involved. Coupled with ADHD, women (and those around them) often find life simply miserable. In Laura McCarthy's article (2009) mentioned above, she cites Dr. Patricia Quinn, developmental pediatrician, author, and ADHD expert, who says that women with ADHD experience more acute PMS symptoms than non-ADHD women. In addition to fatigue, cravings, bloating, cramps, and emotional unevenness, the cognitive abilities of women with ADHD are also impacted, resulting in symptoms like confusion, irritability, forgetfulness, brain fog, and impatience. Sleep problems are also commonly experienced.

If you're prone to anxiety and/or depression, these may worsen during your menstrual cycles, and PMS can cause tremendous difficulty for you. But what happens during pregnancy and childbirth? Do things get better—or worse?

Stretch Marks on the Brain: Pregnancy and Childbirth

Hormones play a huge role in how you feel during pregnancy. With ADHD in the mix, things often get more complicated. Many who stop their ADHD medications upon their doctor's instructions find it very hard to cope, as their symptoms worsen during their pregnancy. (See "Taking Meds During Pregnancy" below.) On the other hand, some women report that their ADHD symptoms improve dramatically and they are relieved that they can manage without their medications. This may be because their estrogen levels rise as their pregnancy progresses, but then symptoms come raging back after childbirth, when hormones drop again. Postpartum depression can become a significant issue, especially if you've been struggling with depression before your pregnancy. Depression is commonly seen in women with ADHD. In addition, caring for a newborn (and possibly other children, often young, with high demands) means sleep deprivation and more stress, which worsens attention, focus, mood, and concentration.

Taking Meds During Pregnancy

You might be wondering if it's okay to take stimulant medications while pregnant. Since there are no studies out there on humans (it's an ethical dilemma to give medications to pregnant women in order to study safety and efficacy), this is a discussion you'll need to have with your health care provider. Most stimulants are classified "category C" teratogens, which means they should only be used when the risk posed to the mother by not taking them outweighs the risk of taking them for the fetus. All women worry about the health of their unborn child. And though there are no studies to show the effects of prescribed stimulants taken during pregnancy, your doctor will want to ensure a healthy pregnancy and healthy baby, so any medication taken during pregnancy can be a source of concern. Do discuss your options with your doctor so you can make the safest choices possible. In the article "Can a Woman with ADHD Take Stimulant Medication While Pregnant" on its FAQ page, the National Resource Center on ADHD says this:

> To date, the effects of stimulants during pregnancy have only been studied in animals, where defects were seen in the offspring when the mothers were given very high doses of the stimulants. The doses of stimulants given to animals for these studies have been 41 [times] and 12 [times] the usual human dose. The literature contains individual case reports of women who have taken stimulants during their pregnancy and, clinically, there have been many other women who have taken stimulants and have had normal babies.

It can be a dilemma for you if you've depended on stimulants to get through your day. Ultimately, it's up to you and your doctor to make the decision whether to continue or stop taking them. It might help to remember that pregnancy is a temporary state and that soon you'll be able to resume your medication regimen.

Now that you've gotten through your pregnancy, you are probably hoping the worst is over. But...surprise! Other life and hormonal changes can also affect your symptoms.

Perimenopause, Be Gone!

Now that you're a bit older, perhaps you've settled into a stable routine at work and in your home life. But don't forget that your body is constantly changing, even now. Along comes perimenopause, which creates new problems to deal with. This is also a time when clinicians often see women for the first time as they seek help for their out-of-control ADHD symptoms. Maybe you, at middle age, are finding that your symptoms have gotten worse, too. It's confusing because life appears to have settled down, but your hormones didn't get the memo! This is also a time when women begin wondering if they might have early onset dementia, as word retrieval and short-term memory often become worse along with other ADHD symptoms. One of the key differences between hormone-related memory problems and dementia is that with dementia you no longer remember how to do things you've done many times before, like driving to the market or following a favorite recipe. With dementia, there might also be permanent changes in mood and personality, whereas with hormonal memory problems, your moods are transient, and you often come back to baseline. In a study of 117 middle-aged women, published in the *Journal of the North American Menopause Society*, researchers Weber, Rubin, and Maki (2013, 511) concluded that "decreases in attention/working memory, verbal learning, verbal memory, and fine motor speed may be most evident in the first year after the final menstrual period." There is no doubt that women in their forties and fifties tend to experience aggravated issues of memory loss.

So it's true that such changes take place for many women but perhaps more so for the woman with ADHD who already struggles with memory-related symptoms. In a study published in the July 2012 issue of *The Journal of the North American Menopause Society*, University of Rochester researchers Weber, Mapstone, Staskiewicz, and Maki confirm that hormone-related memory loss is not associated with later dementia. In fact, they did not find any connection between middle-aged women who report memory problems and women who later develop serious memory loss.

If you've noticed your memory worsening, thinking you have early-onset dementia, this study should put your worries to rest. According to the Mayo Clinic's (n.d.) article "Early-Onset Alzheimer's: When Symptoms Begin Before Age 65," "Of all the people who have Alzheimer's disease, only about 5 percent develop symptoms before age 65." Of course, if your memory suddenly changes significantly, and you have concerns, do discuss this with your health care provider. But all in all, changes in memory are common during perimenopause. This, combined with ADHD, can be upsetting because there is already a baseline of difficulties that is now exacerbated by changes in hormones.

Along with these cognitive changes often come mood swings, sadness, irritability, chronic worrying, and sleep disturbances. Your periods become erratic due to more hormonal changes. Excessive bleeding (flooding), called *menorrhagia,* can leave you anemic, adding to fatigue and brain fog to the point where you might feel that you can no longer cope. All this can contribute to the possibility that your ADHD meds are no longer working optimally.

Perimenopause, the stage before menopause, is a time when your estrogen levels decrease. According to Dr. Patricia Quinn's book *100 Questions & Answers About Attention-Deficit/Hyperactivity Disorder (ADHD) in Women and Girls,* "It is a time often associated with mood changes and the onset of depression in some women who have had no previous history of the disorder" (2011, 136). And now, your hormones change yet again as you enter menopause. How does that affect your ADHD?

She's Homicidal, Weepy, and Sweaty: Don't Mess with Her

As you enter the next stage of your life, menopause, you'll find that this, too, typically affects your ADHD symptoms as your estrogen continues to decrease and new stressors enter your life. Perhaps you are now caring for elderly parents or are experiencing medical problems associated with advancing age. In addition to the hot flashes, depression, and sleep disturbances that many experience, women often have issues with mental clarity, word retrieval, and memory loss, all of which can greatly aggravate someone who already has ADHD. Short-term verbal memory often worsens as you find yourself searching for the right word or immediately forget a person's name after you're introduced. These, of course, are also symptoms of ADHD, but they only worsen as your estrogen level becomes depleted, making you question your ability to stay on top of things. In her article "The Hormonal Influences on Women with AD/HD" (2002, 97), Patricia Quinn, MD, points out that doctors typically increase a woman's stimulants during menopause to treat these symptoms, but with little benefit. As women complain of worsening symptoms, what really needs to be addressed is their change in hormones. "Several studies have now documented that women receiving hormonal therapy performed significantly better on cognitive testing....[W]omen with menopausal symptoms who received hormone replacement therapy improved verbal memory, vigilance, reasoning, and motor speed....[The therapy] was also shown to enhance both short- and long-term memory and the capacity for learning new associations."

So, though your life may seem to be less complicated than in earlier years, your biology is actually making life even more challenging. As you pass from menopause into postmenopause, these problems continue as your estrogen levels become more and more depleted. But don't despair! There are ways to work around all of this.

You Are More than Your Hormones!

We'll soon discuss specific solutions for dealing with hormone stressors at each stage of a woman's life. Before we do that, though, let's look at some general suggestions for dealing with hormonal stressors, regardless of which phase you are in:

- Find an OB/GYN who is familiar and/or sympathetic with ADHD who can prescribe hormonal treatments.

- Work closely with whoever is prescribing your ADHD meds to tweak dosages or make changes as needed.

- Cut back on caffeine and sugar.

- Start an exercise routine!

There is no reason to suffer unnecessarily. You will need to be proactive in getting help and making changes in your lifestyle in order to feel your best.

There are solutions to consider that will help you or those you love as you enter each new phase of hormonal change. Let's start with how to help your teenaged daughter as she enters puberty.

Support for Tweens 'n' Teens

Earlier in this chapter, you learned how your daughter's changing hormones are probably contributing to her worsening ADHD symptoms. Now let's look at some ways to help her through these difficult ups and downs that she experiences each month. First, teach her how to track her periods so that she can prepare for changes in her mood and cognitive abilities. (See http://ADDconsults.com for relevant apps that she can download onto her smartphone.) Try searching iTunes or other online services using search terms such as "period tracking." Once she has a better handle on her cycles (though it can take years until her cycles become regular), she can then begin to plan around them. For example, if she knows she has a big school project or exam coming up, have her work and study at times when she is feeling good and is mentally at her best. Projects can be tackled well before they are due in order to avoid the hormonal seesaw. This isn't an easy feat, as most students with ADHD tend to procrastinate and complete their work just as the deadline looms over their heads. But with good planning and support, it's possible to get into better homework habits. This is when she can use extra support from you, her dad, or a helpful tutor or coach. A sympathetic teacher might also modify her deadlines, giving her a bit of leeway. And if she qualifies for an IEP or 504 (special education services and accommodations), it may be necessary to address this problem there. As much as you want to help your daughter, you'll also need to go easy on her right before and during her period, but do educate her on how her hormone fluctuations affect her ADHD symptoms.

Relax your expectations and demands, and understand your daughter's outbursts without taking them personally. That's not to say that outbursts are acceptable if they are hurtful or disruptive. Show her more effective ways to deal with her stress and offer support. You can do this by helping her with balance, structure, and awareness—for instance, by showing her how to balance schoolwork with free time and schedule her days to reduce stress, and educating her on the impact her ADHD might have on different areas of her life. You can also teach her (and model) the basics such as adequate sleep, good nutrition, exercise, and avoiding excessive sweets. All these tips will help with adolescence in general, but here are some tips for dealing with the added burden of ADHD coupled with PMS.

PMS: Potentially Manageable Symptoms!

Timing is everything if you're a woman with ADHD *and* PMS. Get to know your body's rhythms, and pace yourself. Now is *not* the time to make any major life decisions. This can be challenging if you happen to be impulsive, but it's important to save those decisions for when you are feeling more balanced. And try to avoid emotionally charged discussions until after PMS. Better to wait to schedule that chat with your boss about a raise! Just as I mentioned for adolescents, mark in your planner or calendar when your next period is due and keep track so that, if at all possible, you don't schedule stressful meetings, work projects, or other important obligations during those times. Keep your work schedule as light as possible and allow for extra downtime. In addition to timing, communication can also go a long way to maintaining your relationships during this time when you are not "yourself."

Tell 'Em How You Feel!

Let your family and close friends know how your PMS impacts your behaviors and how it ties into your ADHD—and when you're about to experience PMS! If by chance you do or say things that affect them during those times, don't hesitate to explain yourself. You are still responsible for your actions, but it always helps to explain why your behavior is "off." Even children should be informed when Mommy is having a bad day, so they know it's not their fault. Your partner needs to know as well so that you can plan how to work together as a team during these stressful, uncomfortable times.

Your Doc as Your Ally

More than ever, you need a good working relationship with your health care providers. It's ideal if your OB/GYN communicates with your general practitioner, your psychiatrist, or whoever prescribes your ADHD meds so that the meds can be tweaked if necessary. ADHD meds may need to be changed in dosage or type, or you may want to add (or increase) an antidepressant if you find you're struggling more with depression while you're premenstrual. After consulting with your ADHD doc, your gynecologist might suggest hormone replacement therapy. Whatever the case, it's best to have a team in place to help you with your medications when your hormones are making your ADHD symptoms worse. For most women, dealing with the usual hormonal shifts and/or PMS is challenging enough, but some women opt to take the next leap and have a little bundle of joy, who will bring new hormonal shifts and demands.

Pregnancy and Childbirth

Yay! You've found that you're expecting! As you dream of baby clothes and baby names, your body changes in many ways, and so do the effects of your ADHD. Hopefully, you'll have some relief of symptoms during the latter part of your pregnancy, but if that's not the case, here are some suggestions to help you manage your ADHD.

To Medicate or Not to Medicate?
That Is the Question

First, ask your doctor whether you need to stop your medications. More than likely, the answer will be yes. If your symptoms are so challenging that you need something on board, there are some medications that are safer than stimulants. Some women use omega-3 fish oil, but the jury is still out as to whether it effectively works to decrease ADHD symptoms. Certain antidepressants may be an option, but it is imperative to discuss this with your doctor.

If meds are out of the question, exercise regularly, but get an okay from your doctor first! Swimming is excellent as it gives you a cardiac workout while you enjoy the blissful effects of weightlessness. Prenatal yoga classes can help calm you and offer stretching and other light physical exercises.

Other options worth exploring are neurofeedback, meditation, and brain training programs. Brain training programs are computer-based games developed to improve working memory (the ability to hold, manage, and manipulate information). Though the jury is still out concerning long-term results for most of the programs currently available, they may still be worth trying, as some clinicians report that some clients do indeed benefit from such programs.

Cognitive behavioral therapy (CBT) is also an excellent option, as is working with an ADHD coach. CBT is a psychotherapeutic treatment that helps you change how you think about things and how you react to them. Among other things, it offers pragmatic tools for dealing with disorganization, distraction, and emotional responses to everyday situations, such as family life, work, and relationships. A coach will help you set up strategies, hold you accountable, and keep you on target so you can get tasks and projects done. And even if you feel you don't need it, ask for outside support, especially if you have other children at home. This is even more important once your baby is born, and you need an extra hand.

Help for Working Moms

If you're a working mom and feel overwhelmed and unable to manage your responsibilities effectively, consider working with an ADHD coach, which can make all the difference in the world to help you stay organized and meet deadlines. Or, if this is not feasible, you may want to consider taking a leave of absence or cutting back your hours.

If you have other children, getting help gives you the opportunity not only to get some needed rest, but also to spend one-on-one time with each child before and after the new baby arrives. This is not the time to be Superwoman. Relinquish certain home responsibilities to your partner, or simply let go of any high standards you might be carrying. Bring in someone to clean the house every week or two. Ask a friend or neighbor to help you with carpooling your other children to activities. Cut back on your obligations. Cooking seven nights a week can be too much; getting carryout or going out for dinner can give you a much-needed break. Your number one responsibility is to stay healthy for your sake and the sake of your unborn child and the rest of your family. Household chores and other responsibilities will have to take a backseat for a while. And don't forget to take time away with your partner so you can simply relax and be pampered. A dinner out once a week or once a month without children will make all the difference.

But pregnancy isn't the only time your body goes through a major change. As you get older, your hormones get cranky yet again, as you transition into your forties and fifties.

Perimenopause: Creeping Toward "The Change"

Your body will change as you age. That is inevitable. But knowing what to expect and bringing your awareness to the changes can make all the difference. Just as with PMS, you'll need to be in close communication with your health care providers so that your medication regimen works optimally for you. You may need a change in dosage and an additional medication should you need help with the depression and/or anxiety that sometimes comes with perimenopause. Some women find relief with antidepressants or an increase in stimulant (and/or antidepressant) dosage, as symptoms warrant. You will likely have physical ups and downs due to hormonal changes as well as another potential roller-coaster ride with your ADHD symptoms. It's helpful to understand that your hormones are the reason for the increase in your ADHD-related difficulties.

And once you're in perimenopause, menopause is not that far behind. Again, hormones continue to affect your memory and physical well-being.

Menopause: You Can Switch from "Pause" to "Play"

You might be dreading this next phase of hormonal changes. You've probably heard horror stories of worsening memory and mood and unpleasant physical changes. But don't give up hope. It's not all doom and gloom! In fact, many women report a feeling of overall well-being as they move from perimenopause into menopause. Moods begin to stabilize as estrogen levels out. Many find that anxiety, depression, and other common symptoms of perimenopause improve during menopause. Though certain symptoms do seem to improve during menopause and postmenopause, women with ADHD often find that their cognition and word retrieval are still problematic. Other ADHD symptoms, such as those seen in perimenopause, do continue. Your doctor might suggest increasing your ADHD medications, but again, the main culprit is your estrogen levels, which during this time have dropped significantly. Some find relief with hormone replacement therapy, which may somewhat improve cognitive functioning. In her article "Hormonal Influences on

Women with AD/HD," Dr. Patricia Quinn (2002, 99) states that adding a selective serotonin reuptake inhibitor (SSRI)—a type of antidepressant—can be helpful with mood but also in enhancing the effects of your stimulant medication. She also says that some women might need stimulants plus SSRIs plus estrogen replacement when symptoms get worse with monthly cycles or with menopause. And "estrogen plus stimulants may be necessary to address perimenopausal depression and the cognitive dysfunctions that accompany menopause." But again, it's imperative that you discuss these options with your health care provider.

All in all, understanding how your body is changing, and becoming aware of these changes, can make a big difference in how you feel and help you learn to be proactive in taming your ADHD symptoms. Anxiety over normal changes will make your symptoms worse. Know that you are not going crazy, that you are most likely not developing dementia, and that most of the physical and emotional symptoms will improve. Exercise, challenging mental activities, good sleep habits, and avoiding alcohol and smoking will all help with cognitive symptoms.

Try to lighten up on yourself and enjoy this time in your life. You may have the freedom now to travel and explore new interests. Certain changes come with the territory of aging, so consider adjusting your schedule and lifestyle. And don't forget the benefits of hiring a coach during this new transition in your life.

Yes, there are challenges as your hormones change, but there are positives as well. With maturity often comes a sense of calmness. You're now more stable in many areas of your life and have come to a stronger sense of self. If you've worked through many of your ADHD-related issues, such as low self-esteem, then you will hopefully have learned strategies and compensations for the cognitive changes you might be experiencing now. Remember, not all women have a difficult menopause—and whether one has ADHD or not, some cognitive changes are apt to happen. And now, your non-ADHD female friends and relatives who are also going through these hormonal changes might get an idea of what you've been struggling with all along!

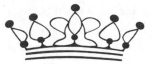

CHAPTER 10

Working Hard at Working

I quit a job once after only four days. Fresh out of graduate school with a brand-spanking-new MSW degree under my arm, I took a job at a foster care agency. I was worried about not knowing the ropes, the laws, or much of anything, and I was terrified that first day of work. My supervisor started me off with an easy assignment: conducting intake interviews over the phone…in a large room…with ten other workers. I'll bet you can see where this is going. I heard every click of the phone, every chair shuffling, and every paper rustling. I thought I was going to go out of my mind because I could not filter out the sounds. I quit because I couldn't make out what the person on the phone was saying, not because the work was too hard or because I didn't understand what was needed of me.

Back then, I had no clue what ADHD was, let alone that I had it. So, of course, it never occurred to me to ask for accommodations. I have heard countless similar stories from women with ADHD when it comes to workplace challenges. Women with ADHD have to work ten times harder than women without ADHD just to meet baseline expectations in the workplace. Picture being on a team of divers tasked with documenting a shipwreck, and you're the only one without an air tank. That's what it's like for the woman with ADHD. Your job includes all the usual workplace expectations like being on time, multitasking, scheduling, prioritizing, organizing, staying focused, and developing and maintaining excellent relationships with coworkers and clients. How do you do it? Just keep swimming! It's exhausting and somewhat terrifying, but those are the rules of the game if you want to play.

Now, this assumes that you've already run the gauntlet of career choices and found one that is a fit. Finding one's life path is challenging enough for those without ADHD, but add a potentially disabling condition to the mix and the choices are greatly diminished. The important thing is to use strategies to help you manage the non-ADHD-friendly aspects of your job. This chapter will address what those are and how to get beyond them. Let's look first at the non-ADHD-friendly aspects of work.

The Usual Suspects: ADHD Symptoms and Work

ADHD follows you everywhere, from home straight to your desk at work. Your symptoms at work simply cause their own unique problems and impact your clients, coworkers, and boss. Getting to work on time can also create anxiety and tension, as well as conflict with your boss. Struggling to keep up with schedules, business meetings, and phone calls can impact how successful you are at carrying out your work duties and also cause friction with other staff members. Other challenges include distractions, such as people talking and phones ringing, that impede your ability to focus, and fluorescent lighting, which can make it hard to concentrate. Finding the right environment to work in successfully is hard, but harder yet is figuring out the right career for you.

Playing Career "Twister"

Everyone wants a job they love and excel at, but your ADHD and past experiences, especially all the years you lived undiagnosed and untreated, can lead you to make poor career decisions. As a result, you may even land a job that you hate and that is also not ADD-friendly. You may contort yourself into the position in an effort to conform and play the game, but holding that position can be a setup for failure and stress-related health issues, especially if you do so for a long time. If you received poor grades in school, you probably went into adulthood with low self-esteem and a fear of failure. Even if you excelled in school, you might have worries about finding a job that fits, knowing how hard you needed to work to stay afloat as a student.

Many women with ADHD are underemployed and underpaid because they are afraid of taking the leap into a job they fear might be too difficult for them, resulting in many unhappy years stuck in dead-end, boring, or stressful jobs. And even if you land that job you had always hoped for, your ADHD can hit you squarely between the eyes. Even in a job you love, your unmet ADHD needs can cause many hardships, transforming otherwise wonderful employment into the job from hell. And unlike school, where you can usually get support from your teachers and the disabilities department, your boss and coworkers might not have the same empathy and desire to see you succeed. Not only do you need to think about all the things that go into the right choice of career, but once you land that dream job, you'll need to make another big decision: do you disclose your ADHD or not?

Whom Do You Tell? The Art of Disclosure

If you're incredibly lucky, you've found a job that celebrates your strengths and is a good fit for your ADHD. However, many find that their symptoms still create havoc. How do you get help? Do you disclose your

ADHD? Most ADHD experts suggest not even disclosing your ADHD to your employer because, sadly, many will use the information against you. Some may think you are using your diagnosis as a way to avoid certain obligations and may pile even more work on you. Others might not believe ADHD exists and purposely reject your informal accommodation requests. Or they may become critical or dismissive of your difficulties. Some may think that you will not be able to handle the job because they have no real understanding of ADHD and simply see it as a liability rather than a possible asset. If they think it may inhibit good work, you may be asked to leave. There are a lot of challenges in working for people who don't understand or care to help you with your ADHD-related issues. Is it, then, easier to work for yourself, to be your own boss?

To Be...or Not to Be...an Entrepreneur

Many people dream of being their own bosses and having their own businesses. People with ADHD often think big and have incredibly creative ideas. Perhaps you've had thoughts about being an entrepreneur, working your own hours, and developing ideas, products, or services. Is this the right fit for you?

Walking the Wire Without a Net

Remember that, without the pressure of your boss or having coworkers around, you might be more likely to go off task due to the lack of external structure. It may be harder to meet deadlines and attend to all the details, such as administrative tasks of paperwork, bookkeeping, scheduling, and returning e-mails and phone calls. You may have many ideas but no solid plan to implement them; when a new idea hits, you're off and running, leaving previous ones to languish in the dust. If you're working from home, chances are you may get distracted by your family members, pets, TV, and computer, as well as all the other things that are at your fingertips, vying for your attention. And if you find yourself backed against the wall, losing the battle to get work done by a deadline or facing important paperwork that's grown like weeds, you might bail out of frustration or jump ship when you become bored.

The Money Pit

Managing the finances can also be a huge pitfall. Adults with ADHD (not just women) are prone to mishandling money due to impulsivity or an inability to handle details. Bookkeeping, balancing checkbooks, and paying bills can be especially hard due to the challenges people with ADHD face with executive functioning, procrastination, avoidance, and difficulties with details. That doesn't mean you should avoid going into business for yourself. In fact, many of the most successful entrepreneurs have or are thought to have ADHD. For example, best-selling author, entrepreneur, and marketing genius Seth Godin has ADHD, as does David Neeleman, founder and former CEO of JetBlue Airways. What's important is to have plans in place to support you so that you can thrive being on your own.

Just Keep Swimming...

If you are that tankless diver mentioned at the beginning of this chapter, there are a number of tricks to help you keep breathing in the workplace— even if you don't have an air tank. Let's explore some solutions to help you find success in the workplace, whether you work for someone else or are a self-employed entrepreneur.

Clutter Bug DDT

Don't despair! You can keep your work area clean and "just tidy enough." Keep that terrifying swarm of clutter at bay by setting up an efficient filing system and develop a routine for getting your paperwork done, such as setting aside a specific time each day to handle paperwork. Use the same system that works for you at home. If you need to see your papers and files, use an open filing system instead of an enclosed one. Dedicate time each day to tidying up your workspace and include your "tidy up" time in your planner. This could be the first or/and last ten minutes of your workday. Make it a daily routine. Another important routine? Make sure you look at your planner first thing when you arrive at work.

Making Paperwork Work for You

Don't have a meltdown over paper piles. They can be tamed! Get into the habit of taking care of paperwork as soon as you touch it. Set up a two-level tray and label the trays "Do Today" and "Do Later." Put papers that cannot be taken care of immediately into the Do Today tray. Allot ten minutes at the end of your day to taking care of the Do Today papers. Review the Do Later papers at the end of each week. Delegate or toss any paperwork that realistically you aren't going to do. Consider bartering tasks with coworkers. For example, ask them to handle the paperwork in exchange for taking on phone duty.

Keep the Horse from Going Back to the Barn

You still need some tricks up your sleeve to keep you afloat and organized at work. Here are a few more.

Ask your boss and coworkers to put verbal task requests and communications into an e-mail and send them to you. This way, you won't have to remember all the details, and you'll have those trusty visual cues to keep you on task. The added bonus is that you'll have a record of the requests/communication that you can keep in a special "to do" folder in your e-mail program.

Another helpful idea is to keep a short to-do list for each day and tape it to your desk or wall to keep it visible. (Remember, out of sight is out of mind for the ADHD brain.) Ask your boss to break down large projects into smaller, doable tasks. For repetitive but complicated tasks, write down the steps on index cards and post them in a visible place.

Antidistraction Action

There are lots of ways to manage the many distractions at work. Here are just a few ideas to get you started, but perhaps you can come up with more on your own:

- If possible, switch your work hours so you can come in early or leave late, which will allow you to add exercise time into your day. A brisk midday walk will energize you, bring back your focus, and get you through the afternoon.

- Use noise-canceling headphones to mask distracting sounds with classical music or nature sounds, or wear earplugs if you don't need to interact a lot with staff or customers.

- Use the work library or meeting rooms for extra quiet space when you need to concentrate.

- Turn off your phone ringer and e-mail notification signals when you're in the middle of an important project that demands your full attention. Turn off your e-mail program altogether if you're prone to obsessively checking e-mail.

- Put a "Working Under Deadline: Please Come Back Later" sign on your door or cubicle, or purchase a cardboard clock with movable hands that says, "Will be back at…"

- Set up your chair so that it faces away from foot traffic or other distractions, or if possible, ask for a private office.

- Take frequent breaks to stretch your legs.

- Use a voice recorder for meetings so you can refer back to what was said should you lose focus during a meeting.

- Use a white-noise machine to block out distractions—but only if it isn't a distraction to those around you. It's always best to ask.

Great! Now that you've got some tools for handling the distractions, you're on your way to mastering time management.

No Longer a Slave to Time!

Don't let your ADHD symptoms get the best of you. Just like at home, there are lots of solutions to help you stay on track at work so that you can stay on top of your game:

- Schedule your most challenging work for when you are your sharpest.

- Buddy up with a coworker to get to work on time by sharing a ride.

- Compete with yourself or others to get to work on time.

- Time yourself in the morning to get to work fifteen minutes (or more) early, then work on the details that you might be behind on.

- Ask for flextime. If mornings are tough for you, see if you can come in late and stay late.

- If you have trouble getting up in the morning, subscribe to a service that offers wake-up calls (check online).

- Explore apps and other technology that will help you better manage your time.

- It's important to get help for your ADHD: if you are taking meds, make sure they are working optimally. Find ways to relieve stress—exercise, meditation, good nutrition, and restorative sleep are essential.

- Working with an ADHD coach is invaluable. A coach can help you set up strategies to get you to work on time, manage short- and long-term projects, and handle paperwork and clutter.

These are all great tips to help you find success at work. But what do you do if you can't even decide what sort of job is a good fit for you?

Spinning the Career Bottle

Finding the right job or career takes some deep thought. It can be tough to choose something you are both passionate about and good at. Author and ADHD expert, Wilma Fellman, MEd, author of *Finding a Career That Works for You: A Step-by-Step Guide to Choosing a Career* (2006), has written extensively about careers for men and women with ADHD. She doesn't state which careers are best, but to help *you* find the right match, she suggests that you learn (1) more about yourself—your interests, challenges, strengths, and preferred style of working (for example, physical or sedentary; a job that requires you to think on your feet or one that allows for quiet reflection)—and (2) more about different types of jobs *before* you take on a specific position or career. Simply stated, she reinforces the importance of choosing a career that works for you!

If you find a career you love, your passion will shine through, energizing and motivating you. You'll be leading more with your strengths than your challenges, though you will still need to figure out accommodations for your ADHD. Though typically hyperactive folks seek high-stimulation jobs like police work, emergency room support, or sales, someone else with ADHD may do well as an accountant because she loves numbers, hyperfocuses, and finds deadlines extremely helpful for keeping her on task. Others who thrive in calm environments might seek out careers in writing, research, or computers. Or those same folks might still be drawn to high-stimulation careers because of their interests and skills. Whatever you choose, even if it seems like a mismatch, you need to figure out how to make it work for you.

To help you decide on a career, think about your lifelong dreams. Perhaps you envisioned being a physician because you like to help people, but realize that ten-plus years of higher education is not something you can emotionally or financially handle while managing your ADHD. If the idea of sitting in a classroom for many more years is too unsettling, think of other health care jobs or helping professions that better suit you and that don't require such a rigorous training schedule. But remember, lots of people with ADHD get through medical school. Sometimes passion about the subject matter can help drive the focus necessary to handle demanding academic material.

Tap Your Resources

Ideally, seek out a career counselor with expertise in working with ADHD or other invisible disabilities. To find such a person, contact your state Department of Vocational Rehabilitation for offices near you. Fellman (2006), in *Finding a Career That Works for You*, also suggests visiting job sites and shadowing people to experience firsthand what the job or career entails. ADHD coaches are now beginning to seek out specialized training to help adults searching for career support. You may want to find a coach with this unique background. See http://ADDconsults .com for more information on this type of coaching. Career counselors are trained to help you learn more about your personality, style, strengths, and challenges. Do take advantage of this wonderful resource. Understanding what sort of job is a good match for you will potentially save you from a lifetime of boredom, depression, anxiety, stress, and more.

Honor the "Active" in Hyperactive

If you're the hyperactive/impulsive subtype, you may crave stimulation and movement and be drawn to jobs that require that sort of activity, such as hospital emergency room worker, news reporter, police officer, firefighter, salesperson, preschool or elementary school teacher, performer, or independent contractor. That doesn't mean you can't handle a job that is less physical, but if you do, be sure you have physical outlets during the day to help you stay calm and focused. *Fidgets*—things you can manipulate in your hands, such as stress balls—are helpful. Many women who are hyperactive find that jobs in the military suit their need for structure and accountability.

Inattentive Doesn't Mean Boring!

If you are a woman with inattentive-subtype ADHD, you might crave a quiet, reflective type of job, but that doesn't mean you are limited to a desk job. You might enjoy doing fieldwork in nature or maybe working in a research lab, working in a library, doing technical work, interior design, or teaching yoga.

On the other hand, plenty of inattentive women feel rewarded working in highly stimulating environments like classrooms and in the performing arts. Such jobs, however, may require extra compensations, such as building in downtime to help replenish your energy. Inattentive women typically still have hyperactive brains and need to be challenged and stimulated, so it's important that you don't fall into the sort of job in which you feel stagnant.

Now you have a better idea of how to find the job to best suit you. Next, you need to determine whether or not to share news of your ADHD with your boss or coworkers—and if so, how much you should tell them.

Tell the Half-Truth and Nothing but the Half-Truth, so Help Me, God

Advocating for your needs without putting your job in jeopardy is certainly a challenge. But should you decide to share your condition with your boss and coworkers, here are a number of tips to keep in mind.

The Law Is on Your Side

There are laws to protect your rights. The Americans with Disabilities Act (ADA) now lists ADHD as a disability. The ADA is a set of federal laws designed to end discrimination in the workplace for people with disabilities and to provide equal employment opportunities. This means that, by law, you might be eligible for special supports if you and your workplace meet certain criteria. The ADA protects workers with disabilities in many ways. Employers (again, if certain criteria are met) must offer accommodations (again, under certain conditions) to level the playing field for you. The accommodations aren't specific but can be things like setting up organizational systems, allowing for flextime, providing checklists, offering visual or auditory cues, and similar helps. You can read more about your rights at http://www.ada.gov.

That's the good news. The bad news is that few people are successful in getting the laws to work in their favor so that they can request—and receive—formal accommodations. Likewise, few are successful in winning employment discrimination cases. Even if you absolutely require and are eligible to receive accommodations, it can be incredibly difficult and expensive to win a case against an employer who refuses to provide them. Because of this, it is best to try to work things out with your boss or the human resources department at your place of employment. In fact, most ADHD experts suggest *not* even disclosing your ADHD, as, sadly, many employers will use the information against you. We have a long way to go to educate those in the workplace so that people with ADHD can be employed successfully. In fact, many adults with ADHD bring so much spark, creative thinking, and tenacity to the job that encouraging them through various means of support can only benefit everyone.

Your best bet is to ask for accommodations informally without sharing your ADHD diagnosis. Use descriptive words to explain your difficulty. Start by telling your boss that your intention is to be really productive and that you are serious about doing your best. For example, "I really want to do a great job, but when coworkers constantly interrupt me to tell me something, I often get derailed and then cannot do my best work. Is it okay if I sit in a different room to work on this project?" Always make requests in a positive way from a position of strength.

Bonus Tips

There are lots of things you can do to make your workplace more ADHD "friendly." Here are some additional tips to help you be successful:

- Ask to meet with your boss on a regular basis to make sure you're on track and to show that you're serious about doing your best.

- Use software like spelling checkers and talking calculators as part of the accommodations you make.

- Use color-coded filing systems.

- Use a vibrating watch with alarms and set them to go off throughout the day as a reminder to stay on task.

- Every Monday, review the week ahead of you and break down larger projects into smaller ones; enter each chunk into your planner and note how much time is needed per step. Review your plan with your boss, if possible.

- Always keep a small notebook at hand so that you can jot down comments and requests so you don't forget.

- For important work-related e-mail, be sure that you have an automatic backup on your computer. You can also send copies to your home e-mail address so you have a backup in case they get lost or deleted. (Do this only if it does not break any privacy rules at work.)

Hopefully these tips will help you both be successful and feel successful as you work for someone else.

Some women, however, have found great relief from the stresses of trying to fit into a specific work culture by becoming entrepreneurs and setting up their workspaces and assignments to accommodate their ADHD. Let's learn a bit more about how they make being an entrepreneur work.

If I Were Queen…

If you're having a hard time fitting into the corporate world, and if you like the idea of being your own boss, have lots of ideas, and are highly motivated, consider starting your own business! I have often seen that those with ADHD have many qualities of the entrepreneur: they're creative, open to new strategies, and willing to take risks. (This is especially true of the hyperactive/impulsive subtype.) But being on your own without any built-in structure can cause problems. What do you do to avoid the many potential ADHD-related pitfalls? In order to be successful, you'll need to find ways to accommodate your ADHD tendencies and symptoms.

Coaches Rule! (in a Good Way)

Before jumping in with a grand business idea, it's a good idea to hire a business coach to help you develop one-, three-, five-, and ten-year plans as well as to hold you accountable for every step of getting there. And working with an ADHD coach is almost a must. Your coach will help you set up systems in order to stay on top of all the things that generally throw you off your game: time management, paperwork, clutter, and so on. If hiring an ADHD coach isn't an option for you due to financial restrictions, then perhaps you might look for a business partner who balances your weaknesses with his or her strengths, and vice versa. Perhaps you are the creative force in the business, while your partner is gifted at handling details like bookkeeping, structure, and management.

If you start your own business, you may work by yourself or with others. Even though you may be working with fewer people than if you worked for someone else (though not always), you still have to figure out how to deal with distractions. Let's look at some ways to do that.

Oh, This Will Just Take a Minute (Three Hours Later...)

Now that you are a business owner, all the responsibilities rest on your shoulders. How do you balance everything—setting goals, staying focused, and managing distractions—while dealing with your ADHD at your home office? Here are a few tips:

- Schedule the things you hate doing and things you like doing in your planner (or other time management device) to make sure both get done daily.

- Use a timer to remind you to get back to "ugh work"—the things you hate to do.

- If you're more productive at night, work late at night until the early hours; or conversely, if you're a morning person, start work very early, as long as that fits into your lifestyle and with the needs of your family.

- Another option is to keep regular hours as though you were working in someone's office. Try to keep your schedule consistent and follow your planner!

- If you're working from home and you have a family, put a sign on your door with your schedule. Discuss ahead of time when it's okay to be interrupted.

- Treat your home like a regular work environment. Have a workspace away from distractions that is equipped with items you need.

- Use white-noise machines to help mask auditory distractions.

- Hire a virtual assistant to handle all the details so you can focus on the main aspects of your business and not get derailed. Focus on your strengths!

- Schedule creative time to develop ideas. You are less likely to be all over the place during the day if you get some "juicy" brainstorming ideas.

- Cover a complete wall with whiteboards and bulletin boards so you can jot down ideas as they come to you, and write short to-do lists to keep you on track.

- Buy a little digital audio recorder, use the memo function on your cell phone, e-mail yourself, or send yourself a voice mail to capture "big" ideas, especially when you're away from your office.

Now that you have some ideas for how to organize your "internal" space, it's time to organize your "external" space so that it works for *you*. Here are some ideas to get you started.

Playing with Your Space

Since you now have more flexibility in where and how you'll work, you'll want to maximize your space and organizational options in order both to be comfortable and to be as productive as possible. I thought that describing my home office and how I set it up to suit me might be helpful, so here goes. Maybe it will give you some ideas for yours.

You Are Now Entering... "The Terry Zone"

When I first started working out of my home, I took a spare bedroom for my think-tank workspace. Since I have *visuospatial difficulties*—meaning a hard time visualizing things—I hired a professional organizer to get me set up and to teach me strategies for keeping my workspace organized. I also hired a decorator who could pull together the room in a way to make it not only attractive but "ADHD friendly" as well. The professional organizer (yes, there are POs who specialize in ADHD!) installed shelves in the closet and organized the space so that it made logical sense: office supplies in one area, binders in another, and so on. Those of us with ADHD usually have the "out of sight, out of mind" syndrome, so she showed me how to take an item, like a brochure, out of its box and fold it over the edge so that I had a visual cue as to what was in the box. My printer, scanner, and fax machines are in the closet, along with professional journals, magazines, and more. The decorator assessed my needs with me, and then helped me choose lots and lots of storage for my books and files. The files are in closed file cabinets: work files in one area of the room, personal files in another. My greatest joy is my stainless steel desk that spans the entire back wall of the room so that I can really spread out. Since I can't picture things in my head, I have no idea where my projects and materials are. I have to be able to *see* my stuff in order to function at my best. With my long table, I can keep many of my important things in plain view.

Manageable clutter is not always a bad thing. For many of us, our creative juices flow when we have visual stimuli prompting us. I have a large bulletin board on the front of the closet door and three smaller ones near that. There are also slanted storage bins on two walls that hold spiral notebooks for all my various projects, along with magazines and journals. Of course, I also have the computer on the desk and lots of lamps along with natural light coming in from two windows. And for me, a comfortable office chair is a must. To remind myself that I need to take breaks, I have a cozy recliner in one corner with reading material next to it. There's also a small sofa to encourage my family to hang out with me when I'm taking breaks or just keep me company by doing a quiet activity while I work.

You might also want to carve out a small space where you can relax and meditate or listen to calming music as you work or take breaks. (For more details on how to prepare such a space, look for the "Terry's ADHD Comfort Zone" section in chapter 11.) Whiteboards, bulletin boards, and flip charts will help you capture your ideas and keep you on track. If at all possible, find a work area that has a door so you can shut out distractions. But if there's simply no space or if your home is too distracting, you might need to consider renting office space elsewhere.

Setting up a workspace is just half the battle. Now that you're your own boss, how do you manage your finances?

Let's Face It—M-M-Money Make$ the World Go Around

Though money management can be a real challenge, there are lots of ways to get around this often tedious, detail-oriented task. Here are some ideas to help you with this often very difficult part of your business:

- Set up automatic online bill payments to cut down on paperwork.

- Consider hiring a bookkeeper or virtual assistant to manage your financial paperwork and bookkeeping, ideally someone who is empathetic and understands your difficulties. Remember the theme I've repeated throughout this book: that getting outside help and accommodations is not a luxury but a necessity.

- Find a business partner who has strengths in this area.

- Open up one dedicated business credit card with a low cap to prevent impulse buying. Only use the credit card for business-related purchases so that there is a "paper trail."

- Open a bank account that offers text or e-mail reminders when your account balance is getting too low.

Money management isn't always easy, but it doesn't have to stop you from being successful. Now that you have the gist of things and are ready to jump in, here are a few more tips to help you on your way.

Bonus Tips

Every day, there are more and more resources out there to help the busy entrepreneur. Below are just a few ideas:

- You can contract out all sorts of jobs—big and small—by using websites dedicated to freelancers such as http://www.elance.com and http://www.odesk.com. You can find bookkeepers, Web and graphic designers, phone support staff, and much more.

- Kids often love to help out a parent. If you are a mom, consider hiring your child to help with filing and other office chores.

- MBA students are often in search of part-time work or even internships. Contact your local college to find eager interns.

Working on your own can be an exciting, satisfying experience. And as long as you have the supports you need, you can truly sail.

Women with ADHD have much to juggle in life, from managing a home and family to enjoying a fulfilling career. Getting the help you need for your ADHD is the key to making it all work. It's not always an easy road, but it is entirely doable as long as you have a good understanding of your ADHD, how it affects you, and what you need in order to make your ADHD work for you.

CHAPTER 11

Putting the Jigsaw Together

It all started with my ninety-year-old stepfather breaking his hip, which required immediate surgery, lengthy rehab, and twenty-four-hour care upon discharge. For three weeks, I was at the hospital nearly every day. I fielded phone calls in the middle of the night, coordinated his care, checked in with doctors, and worked out schedules. I lent support to my stressed and upset eighty-six-year-old mother. My house was full of out-of-town relatives who needed to be fed (most with different dietary needs) and entertained, including twin toddlers who needed constant attention. I also looked after my daughter, who has ADHD and other special needs. Add to that the deadline for this book, and I was really under the gun. Oh, and, of course, I worked as usual.

I can handle this, no problem, I thought. But everyone else's needs came first. The stress built up until my world caved in. I couldn't plan. I was overwhelmed by countless people coming, going, talking—and needing to eat! My stomach ached and I felt nauseated, tense, and overreactive. And the worst part? My old tapes kicked in: *What is wrong with me? Why am I not enjoying my family? Why am I so exhausted?*

Finally, to stay sane, I asked everybody to choose their own meals from a local market, and we used paper goods. I asked my husband to keep the snacks coming. I hired a companion to help with my daughter who, like me, was overwhelmed by the commotion. I retreated into my art and music studio whenever possible to enjoy the quiet solitude or to jam. I couldn't eat with the family, so I waited until they were done and then ate in a quiet corner by myself. I also leaned heavily on my older daughter to set up meals and clean up afterward. Despite the accommodations, it was still hard, but I survived and recovered my self-esteem much faster than I would have in the days before I started my journey into understanding ADHD.

Even when you're well equipped with great tools, stuff still happens. But don't let it drain the life out of you. It's temporary and you will jump back. Having all the tips, tools, and support mentioned in this book can help you get through it and get back to baseline faster, and, hopefully, your self-esteem won't take a beating like it used to. You may live through a crisis, but you don't need to define yourself by this crisis anymore. It can be a relative blip on the radar of life.

Women in our contemporary culture are jugglers by trade: mom, spouse, passionate partner, planner, counselor, cook, bowling buddy, BFF (best friend forever), employee, or entrepreneur, to name a few. Today's woman holds herself to the extremely high expectation that she should be able to do it all and do it with competence, flair, and a triumphant smile. When she doesn't measure up, or can't "keep it up," she internalizes guilt and blame, which leads to depression. So now a woman with ADHD who already struggles with feelings of self-doubt regarding her competence gets to add depression to the list of ways in which she is failing. *Buck up!* she tells herself. *What's wrong with you? Why can't you handle stuff like other women do?* To manage her depression, she may turn to self-soothing behaviors, such as shopping, TV watching, Internet surfing, overeating, or gambling. And then before she knows it, she has another problem—addiction.

This final chapter is devoted to reviewing the pieces of the ADHD jigsaw that we discussed in previous chapters along with a dash of additional insight to help you put your own ADHD jigsaw together.

Terry's Notes

Let's briefly review the main points of each of the chapters so you can refer back to them whenever you get stuck and need a quick memory jog. Think of these as Terry's CliffsNotes to the book:

- ADHD is not an excuse; it's an explanation of your difficulties (chapter 1).

- Ask for help. You are not lazy or incapable, but you do need to reach out for support and accommodations for a real, valid medical condition (chapter 1).

- To help deal with clutter, create a home for everything and lower your expectations. It's okay to have areas of clutter as long as you are "just organized enough" (chapter 2).

- Simplify meals, take shortcuts, and use labels to organize and index cards as guides (chapter 3).

- To manage your time, become best friends with your planner and work with an ADHD coach (chapter 4).

- Simplify your clothes by paring down your wardrobe and developing your own "uniform" per season with color accents. Have a trusted friend help with shopping and organizing your closet (chapter 5).

- If you're a mom, get child-care help at times, even when you're at home. Give yourself a time-out from the kids on a regular basis to prevent blowups and being overwhelmed (chapter 6).

- Keep relationships healthy through ongoing open communication or scheduling weekly meetings, if necessary. Note the meetings in your planner (chapter 7).

- Tame hypersensitivities by becoming aware of what they are and figuring out what calms you down. Know thyself—and make accommodations for your comfort (chapter 8).

- Since hormonal changes impact ADHD symptoms, pay attention and work with your doctor to adjust and adapt your medications as needed (chapter 10).

- To survive at work, accommodate, accommodate, accommodate (chapter 10).

- Optimize treatment: in order for any of these tips to work, you need to have "all systems go" with medication (if prescribed), therapy, coaching, and support (chapter 11).

There are still plenty of ways to make your life easier and to feel your best. You may already be doing some of these things, but perhaps you haven't thought of these other suggestions.

Overcommitment = Over the Cliff

Aside from the obvious factors that contribute to balance, such as getting plenty of quality sleep, rest and relaxation, proper nutrition, and exercise, one of the most important—but also one of the hardest—things to do for a woman with ADHD is learning to say no—and stick to it. Learning to say no will make all the difference in helping balance your life.

Are you a "yes-woman"? "Yes, I'll be happy to bake six dozen brownies for the soccer team." "Yes, I'll work every weekend." "Yes, I'll take Grandma to the beauty shop every Saturday." Overcommitment is common in women with ADHD, and it can lead to last-minute scrambling, stress, chaos, and maybe even resentment, all of which will drag you right down into the mucky whirlpool of imbalance.

Why is overcommitment a common trap for women with ADHD? You may like the stimulation of being really busy and feeling needed. Or perhaps you are a people pleaser and don't want to disappoint, especially because you feel you've failed so many people over the years. Also, like many with ADHD, your sense of time may be somewhat distorted, and you may simply misjudge how long it takes to do things. And finally, if you're impulsive, it's too easy to say yes to all of the requests that come your way, but doing so throws you completely out of balance. Being a yes-woman might earn you points and make you feel good about helping others, but at what expense? Your life probably already feels like one big overcommitment (think of all the laundry piles, unpaid bills, unwashed dishes, unfinished work projects), so why are you offering to take on even more? Want to learn a little secret that will move you out of being overwhelmed and back in control of your time?

The Secret to Avoiding Overcommitment

"Let me think about it and get back to you" is a power-packed little phrase that can save you all kinds of trouble! This gives you the chance to go inward and notice your reaction to the request. Did you quiver and hesitate inside? This might be an indicator that you don't really want to do it. Or perhaps you felt honored and excited? Then, yeah! But even if it's something you'd *like* to do, it may or may not fit with your schedule. Using the phrase above gives you a chance to evaluate the request on all levels, emotionally and practically. It buys you time to help keep you from acting on impulse. You might have a terrible time saying no because you want to please, but this little line can help you take ownership of what you can or are willing to do—and what you can't. If you know you can't or you don't want to do something, say, "I'm sorry I can't help you out with this." This is better than saying, "Sorry, I can't help you out this time" because then that person may just change the date and ask you again! Only say "I can't help you out *this* time" if you really want to do what is being asked of you. Below are some guidelines to help you when you absolutely need to give a firm no to a request:

- Use empathy: "I wish I could help you out, but I can't."

- Bargain: "Even though I can't help you with babysitting this weekend, is there something else I can do to help lighten your load? I'm really good at brainstorming ideas or making phone calls."

- Apologize that you're unable to help, but offer to help find someone who is available and suited to the task.

- Simply say no. Sometimes less is more!

So, how do you say no? Here are a couple of scenarios to illustrate how it might sound:

Teacher: "Mrs. Matlen, can we count on you to help supervise the kids on the bus for our class trip to the zoo? I'm sure the kids will love you!"

Mrs. Matlen: *(thinking, "With my hypersensitivities, there is no way I can handle being on a bus with forty screaming kids. I might just jump out the back window.")* "I'm so sorry, but I can't. Why not ask Sally Sanders?"

Boss: "Janet, I'd like you to join the financial committee. Can you please add that to your calendar?"

Janet: "Sure, I'd be happy to assist in any way I can. Before I add that to my schedule, would you be willing to review our goals with me so we can reprioritize the other assignments on my plate?"

Now you're getting the hang of how to free yourself from outside demands. Next, let's move inward to see how you can take control of the choices you make for your own health and well-being.

Smart Foods

The most basic of personal needs is food. There are a number of foods that either feed the brain or aggravate the symptoms of ADHD. Though the little research that has been done specifically on ADHD and diet has met with mixed results, many health experts agree that food can affect brain functioning in general. In the WebMD article entitled "ADHD Diets" (2012), Dr. Daniel Amen, brain researcher and ADHD expert, suggests eating protein (for example, eggs, poultry) in the morning to improve concentration, cutting back on simple carbohydrates (for example, table sugar), eating more complex carbohydrates (for example, berries), and adding foods rich in omega-3 fatty acids (for example, wild salmon). He also recommends taking a daily vitamin and mineral supplement.

In general, eating certain foods at bedtime can help with sleep—insomnia is a common problem for adults with ADHD. For example, according to the article entitled "Food and Sleep" (National Sleep Foundation 2009), pairing a carbohydrate and protein, such as cheese and crackers or peanut butter and bread, can cause just enough drowsiness to help you fall asleep. In a WebMD article, Lisa Zamosky (2009) states that tryptophan, an amino acid found in turkey and chicken, when paired with a carbohydrate, might also do the trick.

And if you're about to reach for a glass of warm milk to help you fall into a deep slumber the way your mom suggested all those years, you may be interested in learning that, according to a *New York Times* article by Anahad O'Connor (2007), it's been found that there is nothing in the milk itself that induces sleep; rather it's the warmth of the beverage or the sweet unconscious memory of falling asleep as a baby with a warm bottle of milk that helps. Regardless of the research, if it works, and it's safe, try it! Foods can, indeed, make you feel better or worse, but what else can you do to make yourself feel better and bring your life into balance?

Balancing Your Zip with Your Z-z-z-z-z

You can literally wear your body out if you drive it like a motor and don't stop or calm yourself down. But it's challenging to find healthy outlets for your hyperactivity, whether it's your body or your brain that is overactive—or both. For example, unhealthy computer or shopping addictions may temporarily feed your need for stimulation, but such behaviors are unsustainable over time. How do you balance your needs for stimulation *and* relaxation?

High-Stim Fun (in Moderation)

There is a misconception that only those with hyperactive/impulsive type ADHD crave stimulation. Those with inattentive type ADHD may be physically sluggish or prefer quiet activities, but many have hyperactive brains that crave stimulation as well. There are a number of healthy outlets to help you avoid the monotony of boredom.

Many women (as well as men and children) with ADHD find that exercise is one of the most reliable, healthy "nonmedication treatments" to help them unwind and focus. John Ratey, MD—associate clinical professor of psychiatry at Harvard Medical School, ADHD expert, author of *Spark: The Revolutionary New Science of Exercise and the Brain* and coauthor of *Driven to Distraction*—states that "exercise is the single most popular tool we have to optimize our brain function....Exercise not only makes us smarter; it also makes us less stressed, depressed, and anxious" (Matlen 2008).

As important as exercise is, it sometimes seems impossible to get yourself into an exercise routine. So, what do you do? Rely on your ol' trusty planner and write in the days and times you'll be exercising.

Schedules are a hated yet necessary part of managing your ADHD, so consider fitting these activities in as part of your overall "feel good" ADHD treatment:

- Take a walk before bed, if you find that helps calm you down.

- Spend a half-hour in green, outdoor spaces every day. Nature stimulates the brain yet calms one's soul. Kuo and Taylor (2004) have published research showing that this helps ADHD symptoms.

- Many women share that sexual activity helps reenergize and simultaneously tame hyperactivity and impulsivity.

- Music can be a great way to get you going and is a fantastic tool to motivate you to get chores done.

- Hanging out in high-energy environments like coffee shops, concerts, sports events, and such can be great for feeding your need for stimulation.

- Chewing gum is an excellent alternative to smoking and can help with focus and excessive energy or anxiety.

- Fidgets (small, hand-held toys to squeeze or play with) are great tools for discharging hyperactivity while helping with concentration.

On the other hand, you may be searching for activities that will calm you down rather than rev you up. Here are some ideas to consider.

Chill Out, Calm Down, Re-e-e-e-lax

Yes, sleeping is one way to enjoy the relaxation your body craves, but there are more ways than just counting z's to calm your stressed-out body. Two helpful ways are meditation and vacation.

Meditation is known to quiet your body, mind, and soul. You may insist that it's impossible to sit still for twenty minutes a day (though you may be surprised!). If that's the case, try walking or dance meditation; this way, your body can still move, but you'll benefit from the effects of meditation to help calm yourself. Walking meditation allows you to be present in the moment while moving. Dance meditation uses rhythm and movement through expressive dance to reach a sense of awareness.

Yoga, though often avoided by women with ADHD as being too quiet or peaceful, can be extremely effective in slowing you down yet making you feel better. There are lots of different types of yoga practices; perhaps a more active form, like Ashtanga, would be more suited for you. Yoga teaches you how to breathe deeply, which changes your body chemistry and relaxes you.

Regular vacations are *necessary* (another accommodation!) for optimal self-care. But you'll need to find the type of vacation that works for you.

An unstructured trip where nothing is planned (think beach vacations) might be soothing to someone without ADHD, but for those with hyperactive ADHD, it might actually cause more anxiety since you may find it hard to sit still with nothing to do—the boredom factor can kick in. Yet for others with ADHD, especially for the inattentive, the idea of lounging in a quiet area with a good book can be the best salve of all. Building in a balance of activities and rest might make for a more satisfying vacation.

It would be great to be able to just get away whenever stress kicks in, but obviously, that is impossible. However, there are ways to set up a comfort zone in your own home, to which you can retreat whenever you need a place to calm down and/or recharge.

Terry's ADHD Comfort Zone

Very little is written about sensory overload in adults with ADHD, but you know all about it because you deal with being overwhelmed all the time. Consider setting up a "comfort zone" in your bedroom or another quiet area of the house (an extra bedroom would be ideal) where you can settle down when you feel overstimulated, are stressed, or simply need some downtime to recharge. The ideas below for setting up your comfort zone are merely suggestions to stimulate your own ideas, because what is comforting to one person can be irritating and unpleasant to another. Consider each of your senses and what you need to calm them.

Visual:

- Bring the green indoors with plants and flowers. Nature is calming.

- Hang pictures, paintings, or posters of nature or serene settings.

- Look for special lighting that is soothing: full-spectrum or colored lights, rock-salt lights, candles, or simply natural lighting by a window. You might even prefer the womb-like safety of a dark room.

- Install a small aquarium with gentle lighting (the bubbling sound of aquarium filters and aerators is also calming for many).

- Paint the walls a soothing color. Many enjoy a light blue-green that evokes the sea, or go with other colors found in nature.

- Hang posters with inspirational quotes that are meaningful to you.

- Stack art and writing supplies for creative outlets.

Tactile:

- Pile up soft cushions on the floor (or a comfy chair), along with a few body pillows.

- Purchase a small piece of carpeting or some throw rugs.

- Lay down memory foam on the floor and cover with a cushiony mattress topper.

- Toss dozens of pillows to cradle your head, shoulders, and back.

- Choose supersoft blankets and pile them up to cuddle in.

- Use a "Bucky" neck pillow (filled with buckwheat groats) to support and soothe your neck.

- Hang a hammock or sling to adjoining walls (or drop it from the ceiling) and throw in soft pillows.

- Install a floating bed. (See http://ADDconsults.com for a link.)

- Use a swinging chair that hangs from the ceiling or one that has its own stand. (See http://ADDconsults.com for a link.)

- Find a rocking chair to soothe you with its rhythmic movement.

- Have a basket of fidgets and other tactile items to play with.

- Invite your pet dog, cat, or bunny to hang out with you. Petting an animal is a soothing activity.

- Include a favorite stuffed animal: you're never too old to hug a stuffed animal!

Auditory:

- Keep an iPod and headphones handy, loaded with soothing music.

- Stream nature sounds on your laptop or purchase them to download to your iPod.

- Use noise-canceling headphones to block out unwanted sounds.

- Include chimes or a small waterfall fountain, which can be very soothing.

Smell:

- Use aromatherapy; many find it helpful for destressing.

- Place essential oils in a diffuser for a calming effect.

Taste:

- Set up a little tea station.

- Have favorite snacks like chocolate or fresh fruits available in a pretty basket.

Your personalized comfort zone can work for whatever "flavor" of ADHD you happen to have, since both the hyperactive and inattentive need ways to calm down. The key is to design the zone just for you and to only include things that *feel* good to you. And if you have children with ADHD in the house, set up a comfort zone for them as well; let them choose what they'd like in their own comfort zone. Just don't let them take over yours!

Now that you're likely feeling calm enough to fall asleep from reading all of these comforting strategies, let's explore how you can find ways to fall asleep at night. We know that sleep issues are a raging problem for many with ADHD. Here are some tips for dealing with that.

Sweet Dreams

We know that restorative, adequate sleep is imperative for optimal functioning and maintaining equilibrium. Though you may feel you'll never get a good night's sleep short of taking a sleeping pill, try these strategies to help you fall into and stay in blissful sleep.

Since your hyperactive brain rebels just when you need it to shut down at bedtime, one way to tame your thoughts, worries, ruminations, and creative ideas is to journal all of your thoughts and details of the day. Keep a notebook by your bedside and jot away your worries before lights out.

There are other ways to help you fall asleep. You can purchase a special pillow that has special sound technology to lull you to sleep. (See http://ADDconsults.com for details.) White noise or earplugs are common solutions, but others swear by books on tape. Or perhaps your doctor will suggest a specific medication for insomnia. And if none of these options work, consider getting a sleep study done to see if there are underlying medical issues that need to be addressed.

You've done all that you can to make yourself feel your best. But there's still more help out there.

Get Support

Now more than ever before, there are resources available to help women with ADHD. Consider this part of your toolbox for managing your self-care. Allow yourself to reach out for help, to explore your options, and to see that there are hundreds and hundreds of other women, just like you, struggling with ADHD. Here are some suggestions:

- Read books on ADHD. You will find a list of my personal recommendations on my website at http://ADDconsults.com, or search online for "women with ADHD."

- Go to local support groups. CHADD (Children and Adults with ADHD) chapters can be found in most major cities (check their website at http://www.chadd.org).

- Attend local and national conferences: CHADD and ADDA are the largest, but watch for smaller ones, too. Visit http://www.add.org and http://www.chadd.org for upcoming conferences, workshops, and webinars. Visit http://ADDconsults.com for a list of other conferences and webinars.

- Find websites with solid, unbiased information. See http://ADDconsults.com for a list.

- Find communities of women with ADHD Go to http://ADDconsults.com, or see if there are any in your community. If not, why not start your own?

- Talk to family members and close friends who not only understand you and celebrate your strengths but also understand and support your challenges.

Reading books and getting support and information at conferences and in support groups can be incredibly helpful. Sometimes, however, even more specific help is needed in order to stay balanced.

Get the Help You Need

Finding outside help, sometimes even from professionals who understand ADHD and who can help you with various areas of your life, can be a godsend for attaining a more balanced life. Remember that these are accommodations, not luxuries:

- ADHD coach

- professional organizers

- therapist who specializes in ADHD

- tutors for the kids

- babysitters, even if you're at home much of the time

- bookkeepers

- virtual assistants

- administrative or personal assistants

- housecleaners, lawn-maintenance companies

Go to http://ADDconsults.com for links to these resources. If money is an issue, consider bartering services.

All of these are support systems to help you live a calmer, healthier life. Now let's look inward for other solutions.

Taking Your Internal Temperature

Taking your internal temperature will reveal a lot to you, telling you whether you're feeling overly stressed or in a steady state. It's important to understand yourself and what your limits are before you overstretch your capabilities and find yourself in stress mode. Your attitude, self-talk, and perceptions will guide you and steer you back on course. By going inward and listening, you'll learn several things:

- when and how to cut back

- when and how to lower your expectations of yourself, your home, and your family

- how not to compare your situation with those of others

- how to acknowledge that your ADHD is a valid medical condition

- how to see yourself as a capable, competent woman who happens to have an ADHD brain.

By reading this book, you have begun your journey into understanding your ADHD. Hopefully, you've learned a bit more about yourself, how your ADHD has impacted you, and what you can do to make your life better, happier, and more fulfilling. You have armed yourself with information, tips, and strategies—not to get *rid* of your ADHD but to make peace with it. You were born with an ADHD brain, and you will go to your grave with an ADHD brain. Life will always be full of challenges and disappointments. But you can choose to remind yourself of all the inner resources you were born with and have acquired over the course of your lifetime.

You know now that it's okay to reach out and ask for help because ADHD is real, and it creates lots of difficulties for you. You know that getting help is not a sign of weakness, but rather a sign of strength because it shows that you have learned about your needs and what it takes to be successful. You have learned to advocate for yourself. Life isn't just about your challenges but also about your talents and abilities, just as it is for everyone else.

Living with ADHD does make life more difficult, but that's where the tips in this book come into play. Learn to reach out and connect not only with the people who love and understand you but also with your ADHD community—the people who, like you, live with ADHD every moment and who are fully aware of what it takes to get through a day. This will help normalize your experience, and it may even allow you to laugh at your quirks. Remember to go with your strengths, acknowledge your difficulties, and embrace every part of yourself. ADHD is not a death sentence; it's just one small part of who you are.

References

Alloway, T. 2010. *Improving Working Memory: Supporting Students' Learning.* Thousand Oaks, CA: SAGE Publications.

Alvarez, M. 2008. "VA-VA-VA-BOOMER! Hollywood Icon Jamie Lee Curtis Goes Topless for the Cover of *AARP The Magazine* and Dishes on Embracing Her Upcoming 50th Birthday." *American Association of Retired Persons (AARP) The Magazine.* Accessed June 5, 2013. http://www.aarp.org/about-aarp/press-center/info-03-2008/vavava boomer-hollywood-icon-jaime-lee-curtis-goes.html.

Barkley, R. 1997. *ADHD and the Nature of Self-Control.* New York: Guilford Press.

———. 2010. *Dr. Russell Barkley: ADHD Is Not a Gift.* Accessed June 29, 2013. http://www.youtube.com/watch?v=4xpEBE9VDWw.

———. 2011. "The Important Role of Executive Functioning and Self-Regulation in ADHD" (online factsheet, 2). Accessed August 31, 2013. http://www.russellbarkley.org/factsheets/ADHD_EF_and_SR.pdf.

———. 2013. ADHD in Adults: History, Diagnosis, and Impairments (online course). Accessed June 29, 2013. http://www.continuinged-courses.net/active/courses/course034.php.

Biederman, J., S. Faraone, S. Milberger, S. Curtis, L. Chen, A. Marrs, C. Ouellette, P. Moore, and T. Spencer. 1996. "Predictors of Persistence and Remission of ADHD into Adolescence: Results from a Four-Year Prospective Follow-Up Study." *Journal of American Academy of Child Adolescent Psychiatry* 35, no. 3: 343–51.

Bröring, T., N. Rommelse, J. Sergeant, and E. Scherder. 2008. "Sex Differences in Tactile Defensiveness in Children with ADHD and Their Siblings." *Developmental Medicine and Child Neurology* 50, no. 2: 129–33.

Courvoisie, H., S. Hooper, C. Fine, L. Kwock, and M. Castillo. 2004. "Neurometabolic Functioning and Neuropsychological Correlates in Children with ADHD-H: Preliminary Findings." *The Journal of Neuropsychiatry and Clinical Neurosciences* 16, no. 1: 63–69.

Fellman, W. 2006. *Finding a Career That Works for You: A Step-by-Step Guide to Choosing a Career.* 2nd ed. Plantation, FL: Specialty Press.

Ghanizadeh, A. June, 2011. "Sensory Processing Problems in Children with ADHD: A Systematic Review." *Psychiatry Investigation* 8, no. 2: 89–94.

Hallowell, E. "Meet Dr. Hallowell—Biography." Accessed June 12, 2013. http://www.drhallowell.com/meet-dr-hallowell/biography/.

———. 2012. *Dr. Hallowell's Blog*; "Seven Habits of Highly Effective ADHD Adults," blog entry by E. Hallowell, n.d. Accessed June 29, 2013. http://www.drhallowell.com/blog/seven-habits-of-highly -effective-adhd-adults/.

Hallowell, E., and J. Ratey. 2011. *Driven to Distraction: Recognizing and Coping with Attention Deficit Disorder.* Revised edition. New York: Anchor Group.

Halverstadt, J. 1998. *A.D.D. and Romance: Finding Fulfillment in Love, Sex, and Relationships.* Boulder, CO: Taylor Trade Publishing.

Healy, M. 2009. "Tips for Better Time Management." *Los Angeles Times,* Health section, March 9, 1.

Lange, K. W., S. Reich, K. M. Lange, L. Tucha, and O. Tucha. 2010. "The History of Attention Deficit Hyperactivity Disorder." *Attention Deficit Hyperactivity Disorders* 2, no. 4: 241–55.

Kuo, F., and A. F. Taylor. 2004. "A Potential Natural Treatment for Attention-Deficit/Hyperactivity Disorder: Evidence from a National Study." *American Journal of Public Health* 94, no. 9: 1580–86.

Matlen, T. 2008. "Dr. John Ratey Discusses Exercise and ADHD in New Book" (blog). Published March 27, 2008. Accessed December 2, 2013. http://www.healthcentral.com/adhd/c/57718/23174/dr-john-adhd-book/.

Mayo Clinic. N.d. "Early-Onset Alzheimer's: When Symptoms Begin Before Age 65." Accessed November 15, 2013. http://www.mayo clinic.org/diseases-conditions/alzheimers-disease/in-depth /alzheimers/art-20048356.

McCarthy, L. 2009. "Women, Hormones, and ADHD." *ADDitude*, Published Spring 2009. Accessed November 10, 2013. http://www .additudemag.com/adhd/article/5245.html.

National Resource Center on ADHD, FAQ page, "Can a Woman with ADHD Take Stimulant Medication While Pregnant?" Accessed November 14, 2013. http://www.help4adhd.org/faq.cfm?fid=33&tid =97&varLang=en.

National Sleep Foundation. 2009. "Food and Sleep." Accessed December 1, 2013. http://www.sleepfoundation.org/article/sleep-topics/food -and-sleep.

Novotni, M. 1999. *What Does Everybody Else Know That I Don't?* Plantation, FL: Specialty Press.

O'Connor, A. 2007. "The Claim: A Glass of Warm Milk Will Help You Get to Sleep at Night." *New York Times*, September 4. Accessed December 1, 2013. http://www.nytimes.com/2007/09/04/health /04real.html.

Quinn, P. 2002. "Medical Issues for Women with AD/HD: Hormonal Influences." In *Understanding Women with AD/HD*, edited by K. Nadeau and P. Quinn, 86–99. Silver Spring, MD: Advantage Books.

———. 2011. *100 Questions & Answers About Attention-Deficit/Hyperactivity Disorder (ADHD) in Women and Girls*. Sudbury, MA: Jones & Bartlett Learning.

Ratey, N. 2010. "Getting There from Here: Easing Transitions with ADHD," *ADHD Coach* (blog), June 17, 2010. Accessed April 5, 2013. http://chaddcoach.blogspot.com/2010/06/getting-there-from-here -easing.html

Smith, J. 2012. "Steve Jobs Always Dressed Exactly the Same. Here's Who Else Does." *Forbes*. Accessed September 15, 2013. http://www .forbes.com/sites/jacquelynsmith/2012/10/05/steve-jobs-always -dressed-exactly-the-same-heres-who-else-does/.

Solden, S. 2005. *Women with Attention Deficit Disorder: Embrace Your Differences and Transform Your Life*. 2nd ed. Nevada City, CA: Underwood Books.

———. 2007. "ADHD Mom: The Job from Hell." *ADDitude*, October/ November, 1–2.

Weber, M., M. Mapstone, J. Staskiewicz, and P. Maki. 2012. "Reconciling Subjective Memory Complaints With Objective Memory Performance in the Menopausal Transition (abstract)." *Journal of the North American Menopause Society* 19(7): 735–41.

Still, G. 1902. "Some Abnormal Psychical Conditions in Children: The Goulstonian Lectures." *Lancet* 1:1008–1012.

Weber, M., L. Rubin, and P. Maki. 2013. "Cognition in Perimenopause: The Effect of Transition State." Abstract. *The Journal of the North American Menopause Society* 20: 511–17.

WebMD. 2012. "ADHD Diets." Accessed December 1, 2013. http:// www.webmd.com/add-adhd/guide/adhd-diets.

Zamosky, L. 2009. "The Truth About Tryptophan." Accessed December 1, 2013. WebMD. http://www.webmd.com/food-recipes/features/ the-truth-about-tryptophan.

Terry Matlen, MSW, is a psychotherapist, consultant, writer, and coach. She is the author of *Survival Tips for Women with ADHD* and founder of addconsults.com. Matlen has been interviewed by National Public Radio, the *Wall Street Journal*, *Time Magazine*, the *New York Times*, *US News and World Report*, *Newsday*, *Today*, *CBS This Morning*, *The Jane Pauley Show*, *Ladies' Home Journal*, *Glamour*, and others.

Foreword writer **Sari Solden, MS, LMFT**, is a psychotherapist and consultant in Ann Arbor, Michigan, who has counseled adults with ADHD for over twenty-five years. She is the author of the pioneering books *Women with Attention Deficit Disorder* and *Journeys Through ADDulthood*, as well as a prominent keynote speaker at national and international ADHD conferences. She serves on the professional advisory board of the National Association for Adults with Attention Deficit Disorder (ADDA) and was a past recipient of their award for outstanding service by a helping professional. Solden's areas of specialization include women's issues, inattentive ADHD, and the emotional consequences and healing process for adults who grew up with undiagnosed ADHD.

MORE BOOKS *from*
NEW HARBINGER PUBLICATIONS

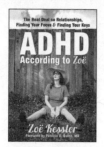
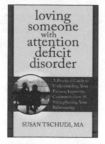
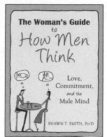
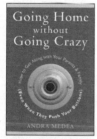
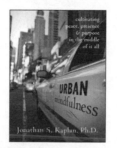
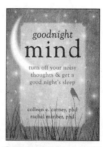

FROM OUR PUBLISHER—

As the publisher at New Harbinger and a clinical psychologist since 1978, I know that emotional problems are best helped with evidence-based therapies. These are the treatments derived from scientific research (randomized controlled trials) that show what works. Whether these treatments are delivered by trained clinicians or found in a self-help book, they are designed to provide you with proven strategies to overcome your problem.

Therapies that aren't evidence-based—whether offered by clinicians or in books—are much less likely to help. In fact, therapies that aren't guided by science may not help you at all. That's why this New Harbinger book is based on scientific evidence that the treatment can relieve emotional pain.

This is important: if this book isn't enough, and you need the help of a skilled therapist, use the following resource to find a clinician trained in the evidence-based protocols appropriate for your problem. And if you need more support—a community that understands what you're going through and can show you ways to cope—a resource for that are provided below, as well.

Real help is available for the problems you have been struggling with. The skills you can learn from evidence-based therapies will change your life.

Matthew McKay, PhD
Publisher, New Harbinger Publications

If you need a therapist, the following organization can help you find a therapist trained in cognitive behavioral therapy (CBT).
The Association for Behavioral & Cognitive Therapies (ABCT) Find-a-Therapist service offers a list of therapists schooled in CBT techniques. Therapists listed are licensed professionals who have met the membership requirements of ABCT and who have chosen to appear in the directory.
Please visit www.abct.org and click on *Find a Therapist*.

For additional support for patients, family, and friends, please contact the following:
Children and Adults with Attention-Deficit/Hyperactivity Disorder (CHADD)
Visit www.chadd.org